NATIONAL ACADEMIES Sciences Engineering Medicine

Applying Neurobiological Insights on Stress to Foster Resilience Across Life Stages

Convened March 24–25, 2025

Janell Payano Sosa, Eva Childers, and
Sheena M. Posey Norris, *Rapporteurs*

Forum on Neuroscience and Nervous System Disorders

Forum on Mental Health and Substance Use Disorders

Board on Health Sciences Policy

Board on Health Care Services

Health and Medicine Division

Proceedings of a Workshop

NATIONAL ACADEMIES PRESS 500 Fifth Street, NW Washington, DC 20001

This activity was supported by contracts between the National Academy of Sciences and Alzheimer's Association; American Academy of Neurology; American Brain Coalition; American College of Clinical Pharmacy; American College of Neuropsychopharmacology; American Neurological Association; American Psychiatric Nurses Association; American Psychological Association; Boehringer Ingelheim; BrightFocus Foundation; California Institute for Regenerative Medicine; Cohen Veterans Bioscience; Council on Social Work Education; Dana Foundation; Department of Health and Human Services' Centers for Disease Control and Prevention; Centers for Medicare & Medicaid Services (75FCMC24P0022); Food and Drug Administration (R13FD005362); National Institutes of Health (75N98024F00001 [Under Master Base HHSN263201800029I]) through the National Center for Complementary and Integrative Health, National Eye Institute, National Institute of Environmental Health Sciences, National Institute of Mental Health, National Institute of Neurological Disorders and Stroke, National Institute on Aging, National Institute on Alcohol Abuse and Alcoholism, National Institute on Drug Abuse, and National Institutes of Health BRAIN Initiative; Office of the Assistant Secretary for Planning and Evaluation (75P00124P00080); and Substance Abuse and Mental Health Services Administration (75S20223P00002); Department of Veterans Affairs (36C24E20C0009); Eisai Inc.; Eli Lilly and Company; Foundation for the National Institutes of Health; Gatsby Charitable Foundation; Harmony Biosciences; Hogg Foundation for Mental Health; Huo Family Foundation; Janssen Research & Development, LLC; The Jed Foundation; Lundbeck Research USA; The Michael J. Fox Foundation for Parkinson's Research; National Association of Addiction Treatment Providers; National Multiple Sclerosis Society; National Science Foundation (DBI-1839674); One Mind; Paul G. Allen Frontiers Group; and Simons Foundation Autism Research Initiative. Any opinions, findings, conclusions, or recommendations expressed in this publication do not necessarily reflect the views of any organization or agency that provided support for the project.

International Standard Book Number-13: 978-0-309-59922-1
Digital Object Identifier: https://doi.org/10.17226/29243

This publication is available from the National Academies Press, 500 Fifth Street, NW, Keck 360, Washington, DC 20001; (800) 624-6242; https://nap.nationalacademies.org.

The manufacturer's authorized representative in the European Union for product safety is Authorised Rep Compliance Ltd., Ground Floor, 71 Lower Baggot Street, Dublin D02 P593 Ireland; www.arccompliance.com.

Printed in the United States of America.

Suggested citation: National Academies of Sciences, Engineering, and Medicine. 2025. *Applying Neurobiological Insights on Stress to Foster Resilience Across Life Stages: Proceedings of a Workshop*. Washington, DC: National Academies Press. https://doi.org/10.17226/29243.

The **National Academy of Sciences** was established in 1863 by an Act of Congress, signed by President Lincoln, as a private, nongovernmental institution to advise the nation on issues related to science and technology. Members are elected by their peers for outstanding contributions to research. Marcia McNutt is president.

The **National Academy of Engineering** was established in 1964 under the charter of the National Academy of Sciences to bring the practices of engineering to advising the nation. Members are elected by their peers for extraordinary contributions to engineering. Tsu-Jae Liu is president.

The **National Academy of Medicine** (formerly the Institute of Medicine) was established in 1970 under the charter of the National Academy of Sciences to advise the nation on medical and health issues. Members are elected by their peers for distinguished contributions to medicine and health. Victor J. Dzau is president.

The three Academies work together as the **National Academies of Sciences, Engineering, and Medicine** to provide independent, objective analysis and advice to the nation and conduct other activities to solve complex problems and inform public policy decisions. The National Academies also encourage education and research, recognize outstanding contributions to knowledge, and increase public understanding in matters of science, engineering, and medicine.

Learn more about the National Academies of Sciences, Engineering, and Medicine at **www.nationalacademies.org**.

Consensus Study Reports published by the National Academies of Sciences, Engineering, and Medicine document the evidence-based consensus on the study's statement of task by an authoring committee of experts. Reports typically include findings, conclusions, and recommendations based on information gathered by the committee and the committee's deliberations. Each report has been subjected to a rigorous and independent peer-review process and it represents the position of the National Academies on the statement of task.

Proceedings published by the National Academies of Sciences, Engineering, and Medicine chronicle the presentations and discussions at a workshop, symposium, or other event convened by the National Academies. The statements and opinions contained in proceedings are those of the participants and are not endorsed by other participants, the planning committee, or the National Academies.

Rapid Expert Consultations published by the National Academies of Sciences, Engineering, and Medicine are authored by subject-matter experts on narrowly focused topics that can be supported by a body of evidence. The discussions contained in rapid expert consultations are considered those of the authors and do not contain policy recommendations. Rapid expert consultations are reviewed by the institution before release.

For information about other products and activities of the National Academies, please visit www.nationalacademies.org/about/whatwedo.

APPLYING NEUROBIOLOGICAL INSIGHTS ON STRESS TO FOSTER RESILIENCE ACROSS THE LIFESPAN PLANNING COMMITTEE[1]

HUDA AKIL (*Co-chair*), University of Michigan
ERIC NESTLER (*Co-chair*), Icahn School of Medicine at Mount Sinai
DEANNA BARCH, Washington University in St. Louis
INDIDA BIRTO, Here's to Life
NADINE BURKE HARRIS, ACE Resource Network
BRIAN DIAS, University of Southern California
EVA FELDMAN, University of Michigan
ANDREW FULIGNI, University of California, Los Angeles
FRANCES JENSEN, University of Pennsylvania
JOHN KRYSTAL, Yale University
HUSSEINI MANJI, Oxford University; Duke University; Yale University; UK Government Mental Health
MICHAEL MILHAM, Child Mind Institute
CATHERINE JENSEN PEÑA, Princeton University
ALEKSANDRA VICENTIC, National Institute of Mental Health

Health and Medicine Division Staff

SHEENA M. POSEY NORRIS, Director, Forum on Neuroscience and Nervous System Disorders
ALEXANDRA ANDRADA SILVER, Director, Forum on Mental Health and Substance Use Disorders
EVA CHILDERS, Program Officer (*until July 2025*)
KIMBERLY OGUN, Senior Program Assistant (*until July 2025*)
CHRISTIE BELL, Senior Finance Business Partner
CLARE STROUD, Senior Director, Board on Health Sciences Policy

[1] The planning committee's role was limited to planning the workshop, and the Proceedings of a Workshop was prepared by the workshop rapporteurs as a factual summary of what occurred at the workshop. Statements, recommendations, and opinions expressed are those of individual presenters and participants; have not been endorsed or verified by the Health and Medicine Division of the National Academies of Sciences, Engineering, and Medicine; and should not be construed as reflecting any group consensus.

Fellow

SHAIKHAH (SHAY) ALSHUAIB, Christine Mirzayan Science and Technology Policy Fellow (*until May 2025*)

Consultant

JANELL PAYANO SOSA, Science Writer

FORUM ON NEUROSCIENCE AND NERVOUS SYSTEM DISORDERS[1]

[1] The National Academies of Sciences, Engineering, and Medicine's forums and roundtables do not issue, review, or approve individual documents. The responsibility for the published Proceedings of a Workshop rests with the workshop rapporteurs and the institution.

HUGH MARSTON, Boehringer Ingelheim (*until May 2025*)
BILL MARTIN, The Janssen Pharmaceutical Companies of Johnson & Johnson
DAVID McMULLEN, Food and Drug Administration
CAROLINE MONTOJO, Dana Foundation
JOHN NGAI, BRAIN Initiative
SANJEEV PATHAK, Acadia Pharmaceuticals
GENTRY PATRICK, University of California San Diego
STEVE PAUL, Seaport Therapeutics
SRI RAMULU PULLAGURA, Foundation for the National Institutes of Health (*starting June 2025*)
KATHRYN RICHMOND, Allen Institute
MARSIE ROSS, Harmony Biosciences
M. ELIZABETH ROSS, American Neurological Association
KATIE SALE, American Brain Coalition
RAYMOND SANCHEZ, Bain Capital Life Sciences
TERRENCE SEJNOWSKI, Salk Institute for Biological Studies
JOAN SERENO, National Science Foundation
SARA SHNIDER, One Mind
DAVID SHURTLEFF, National Center for Complementary and Integrative Health
JOHN SPIRO, Simons Foundation
ALESSIO TRAVAGLIA, Foundation for the National Institutes of Health (*until June 2025*)
NORA VOLKOW, National Institute on Drug Abuse
CHRISTOPHER WEBER, Alzheimer's Association
DOUG WILLIAMSON, Independent Consultant
GARY WILSON, Huo Family Foundation
RICHARD WOYCHIK, National Institute of Environmental Health Sciences
STEVIN ZORN, MindImmune Therapeutics, Inc.

Health and Medicine Division Staff

SHEENA M. POSEY NORRIS, Director, Forum on Neuroscience and Nervous System Disorders
EVA CHILDERS, Program Officer (*until July 2025*)
KIMBERLY OGUN, Senior Program Assistant (*until July 2025*)
CHRISTIE BELL, Senior Finance Business Partner
CLARE STROUD, Senior Director, Board on Health Sciences Policy

FORUM ON MENTAL HEALTH AND SUBSTANCE USE DISORDERS[1]

MARGARITA ALEGRÍA (*Co-chair*), Harvard Medical School
ROSALIE LICCARDO PACULA (*Co-chair*), University of Southern California
CARLOS BLANCO, National Institute on Drug Abuse
W. PERRY DICKINSON, University of Colorado (*representing the American Board of Family Medicine)*
JOEL DUBENITZ, Office of the Assistant Secretary for Planning and Evaluation
RICHARD G. FRANK, Brookings Institution
HOWARD H. GOLDMAN, University of Maryland at Baltimore School of Medicine
KRISTIN KROEGER, American Psychiatric Association
OCTAVIO N. MARTINEZ, Hogg Foundation for Mental Health
BENJAMIN MILLER, Stanford School of Medicine
ZAINAB OKOLO, The Jed Foundation
ANNIE PETERS, National Association of Addiction Treatment Providers
KATHY PHAM, American College of Clinical Pharmacy
JULIE SEIBERT, National Committee for Quality Assurance
RUTH SHIM, University of California, Davis
MATTHEW TIERNEY, University of California, San Francisco (*representing the American Psychiatric Nurses Association*)
HALAEVALU VAKALAHI, Council on Social Work Education
AARON WEINER, Bridge Forward Group; University of Illinois Urbana-Champaign (*representing the American Psychological Association*)

Health and Medicine Division Staff

ALEXANDRA ANDRADA SILVER, Director, Forum on Mental Health and Substance Use Disorders
ADAEZE OKORO-AJUZIE, Senior Program Assistant (*until May 2025*)
SHARYL NASS, Senior Director, Board on Health Care Services

[1] The National Academies of Sciences, Engineering, and Medicine's forums and roundtables do not issue, review, or approve individual documents. The responsibility for the published Proceedings of a Workshop rests with the workshop rapporteurs and the institution.

Reviewers

This Proceedings of a Workshop was reviewed in draft form by individuals chosen for their diverse perspectives and technical expertise. The purpose of this independent review is to provide candid and critical comments that will assist the National Academies of Sciences, Engineering, and Medicine in making each published proceedings as sound as possible and to ensure that it meets the institutional standards for quality, objectivity, evidence, and responsiveness to the charge. The review comments and draft manuscript remain confidential to protect the integrity of the process.

We thank the following individuals for their review of this proceedings:

DAVID ANDERSON, Child Mind Institute
MEGAN GUNNAR, University of Minnesota
TAMAR GUR, The Ohio State University College of Medicine
ISRAEL ROBLEDO, The Michael J. Fox Foundation for Parkinson's Research

Although the reviewers listed above provided many constructive comments and suggestions, they were not asked to endorse the content of the proceedings nor did they see the final draft before its release. The review of this proceedings was overseen by **TRACY L. BALE,** University of Colorado. She was responsible for making certain that an independent examination of this proceedings was carried out in accordance with the standards of the National Academies and that all review comments were carefully considered. Responsibility for the final content rests entirely with the rapporteurs and the National Academies.

Acknowledgments

The National Academies of Sciences, Engineering, and Medicine staff would like to express gratitude to the sponsors of the Forum on Neuroscience and Nervous System Disorders and the Forum on Mental Health and Substance Use Disorders for supporting this workshop and other work of the National Academies; to the speakers whose presentations and remarks informed workshop discussions on the mechanisms of stress and resilience across the lifespan and how that knowledge can inform the development of public health interventions to cultivate resilience; to the planning committee members for their time and effort in the development of the workshop scope and agenda; to Stephanie Eldridge (Spark Street Digital), Tunde Ogunfolaju (Spark Street Digital), and Caset Associates for their support in the broadcasting and transcription of the workshop; to Janell Payano Sosa and Billie Smith-Haffener for their writing and copyediting expertise and contributions, respectively, on this proceedings; and to the additional National Academies staff who provided critical support to the workshop and this proceedings: Christie Bell, Lori Brenig, Samantha Chao, Amber McLaughlin, Alexandra Molina, Marguerite Romatelli, Leslie Sim, and Taryn Young.

Contents

Boxes and Figures

BOXES

FIGURES

Acronyms and Abbreviations

ABCD	Adolescent Brain Cognitive Development
ACE	adverse childhood experience
ACTH	adrenocorticotropic hormone
CalAIM	California Advancing and Innovating Medi-Cal
CBT	cognitive behavioral therapy
CDC	Centers for Disease Control and Prevention
DREADD	designer receptor exclusively activated by a designer drug
fMRI	functional magnetic resonance imaging
HPA	hypothalamic–pituitary–adrenal
IL-6	interleukin 6
NMDA	N-methyl-D-aspartate
NPY	neuropeptide Y
PAAS	Pathways for African American Success
PET	positron emission tomography
PTSD	post-traumatic stress disorder
SSRI	selective serotonin reuptake inhibitor

1

Introduction and Background

Stress is the body's physiological and psychological response to internal and external pressures, challenges, or demands, triggering a complex interplay of hormonal and neurological reactions that influence overall well-being (McEwen and Akil, 2020). Over time, excessive or chronic stress can remodel the brain, disrupting cognitive function, emotional stability, and physical health (Akil and Nestler, 2023; McEwen and Akil, 2020). The detriments of stress have gained considerable attention, with the COVID-19 pandemic underscoring its profound effects on mental and physical health (Akil and Nestler, 2023; COVID-19 Mental Disorders Collaborators, 2021; Saad, 2025; Turner et al., 2023; Zhu et al., 2023). This growing awareness has sparked discussions about its long-term consequences and the crucial role resilience plays in mitigating its harms (Akil and Nestler, 2023).

Resilience—the ability to adapt to adversity—is shaped by biological, environmental, and social factors, and its development varies across individuals (Akil and Nestler, 2023; McEwen and Akil, 2020). While some individuals demonstrate strong coping mechanisms, others remain vulnerable, particularly in times of heightened stress (Akil and Nestler, 2023). Moreover, resilience is not a fixed trait; it fluctuates across the lifespan, influenced by neurobiological mechanisms, early life experiences, and environmental factors (Akil and Nestler, 2023; Nestler and Russo, 2024; Rutter, 1985). A comprehensive understanding of these variations could better inform resilience-building interventions and underscores the need for continued research.

Recognizing the growing effects of stress-related disorders and the need for a deeper understanding of resilience mechanisms, on March 24–25, 2025, the National Academies of Sciences, Engineering, and Medicine's Forum on Neuroscience and Nervous System Disorders, in collaboration with the Forum on Mental Health and Substance Use Disorders, hosted a workshop[1] to explore the current knowledge on stress and resilience mechanisms and provide a foundation for translating research into practical applications. In her opening remarks, Margarita Alegría, chief of the Disparities Research Unit at Massachusetts General Hospital and professor in the Department of Psychiatry at Harvard Medical School, underscored the importance of bridging scientific insights with actionable solutions to foster resilience across diverse populations. Setting the tone for the workshop, Huda Akil, Gardner Quarton Distinguished University Professor of Neuroscience and Psychiatry at the Michigan Neuroscience Institute at the University of Michigan, reinforced this urgency, noting there is still much to learn in the science of resilience. With contributions from leading experts in neuroscience, mental health, and related disciplines—including representatives from academia, industry, patient advocacy, and policy—the workshop provided a multidisciplinary platform to address these pressing issues.[2]

STATE OF SCIENCE ON STRESS AND RESILIENCE

Stress has become a pervasive challenge in contemporary society, reflecting the convergence of rapid societal transformations, technological advancements, and enduring global crises. These stressors have been further compounded by the far-reaching consequences of the COVID-19 pandemic, which acted as a catalyst for what Akil and Eric Nestler, Nash Family Professor of Neuroscience at the Icahn School of Medicine at Mount Sinai, have termed a "second pandemic" (Akil and Nestler, 2023). Akil and Nestler use this metaphor to describe the widespread surge and spread of mental health issues—such as stress, anxiety, depression, and other stress-related disorders—that emerged in the wake of the COVID-19 crisis (Akil and Nestler, 2023).

Most notably, there has been a sharp increase in stress-related disorders, a broad class of conditions shaped by various causes such as genetic predispositions, traumatic experiences, family stress, and even shifts in health. These

[1] To learn more about the workshop, see https://www.nationalacademies.org/event/43074_03-2025_applying-neurobiological-insights-on-stress-to-foster-resilience-across-the-lifespan-a-workshop (accessed May 28, 2025).

[2] The planning committee's role was limited to planning the workshop, and the Proceedings of a Workshop was prepared by the workshop rapporteurs as a factual summary of what occurred at the workshop. Statements, recommendations, and opinions expressed are those of individual presenters and participants; are not necessarily endorsed or verified by the National Academies of Sciences, Engineering, and Medicine; and should not be construed as reflecting any group consensus.

disorders can emerge in diverse forms: from major depression and bipolar disorder to anxiety, post-traumatic stress disorder, and substance use disorders. Within the first year of the COVID-19 pandemic, the world saw 76 million new cases of anxiety disorders and 53 million new cases of major depressive disorders diagnosed, pointing to the profound and ongoing impact of stress on mental and physical well-being (COVID-19 Mental Disorders Collaborators, 2021). While there is a growing perception that the days of the pandemic are over, the current data on its prolonged impact indicate a significant cause for concern. The Mental Health America report of 2024 showed that in the previous year, 23 percent of adults had experienced a mental illness, 13 percent of youth had contemplated suicide, about 20 percent of adolescents (one in five) had a major depressive episode, and 18 percent of adults had a substance use problem (Reinert et al., 2024). The Gallup poll of March 2025 showed that the COVID-19 pandemic disproportionately affected the mental health of specific groups, with certain populations, such as young women between the ages of 18 and 29, experiencing significantly higher levels of stress, anxiety, and other psychological challenges (Saad, 2025).

Stress responses and adaptability vary across individuals, with no single reaction being universal. While some individuals exhibit heightened susceptibility to stress, others demonstrate remarkable resilience (see Figure 1-1). Resilience is broadly conceptualized as the capacity to adapt and maintain positive functioning in the face of adversity (Akil and Nestler, 2023; McEwen and Akil, 2020; Nestler and Russo, 2024). However, resilience in the face of chronic adversity—such as seen in the phenomenon of John Henryism (further discussed in Chapter 3)—can come at a physiological cost, revealing that sustained effort to cope is not always adaptive. In her opening remarks, Alegría emphasized that resilience is not a static trait but rather a dynamic quality that evolves across the lifespan (Akil and Nestler, 2023). She explained that early life experiences, neuroplasticity (the brain's ability to reorganize itself), and the interplay between biological predispositions and environmental influences play significant roles in shaping an individual's ability to respond to stress (Akil and Nestler, 2023; McEwen and Akil, 2020).

For instance, a healthy stress response engages a finely tuned pathway between the brain and endocrine system. Akil said that when stress occurs, the pituitary gland releases a hormone called the adrenocorticotropic hormone (ACTH), prompting the adrenal glands to produce cortisol, which in turn quickly signals a shutdown of ACTH. As she noted, this fast but balanced cycle enables moderate levels of cortisol to enhance synaptic function and neuroplasticity, offering opportunities for learning and coping. On the other hand, Akil stated, excessive stress can lead to an exaggerated or diminished cortisol response, disrupting that balance and reducing the ability to learn and cope. She narrated that on the furthest end of the spectrum, chronic stress—

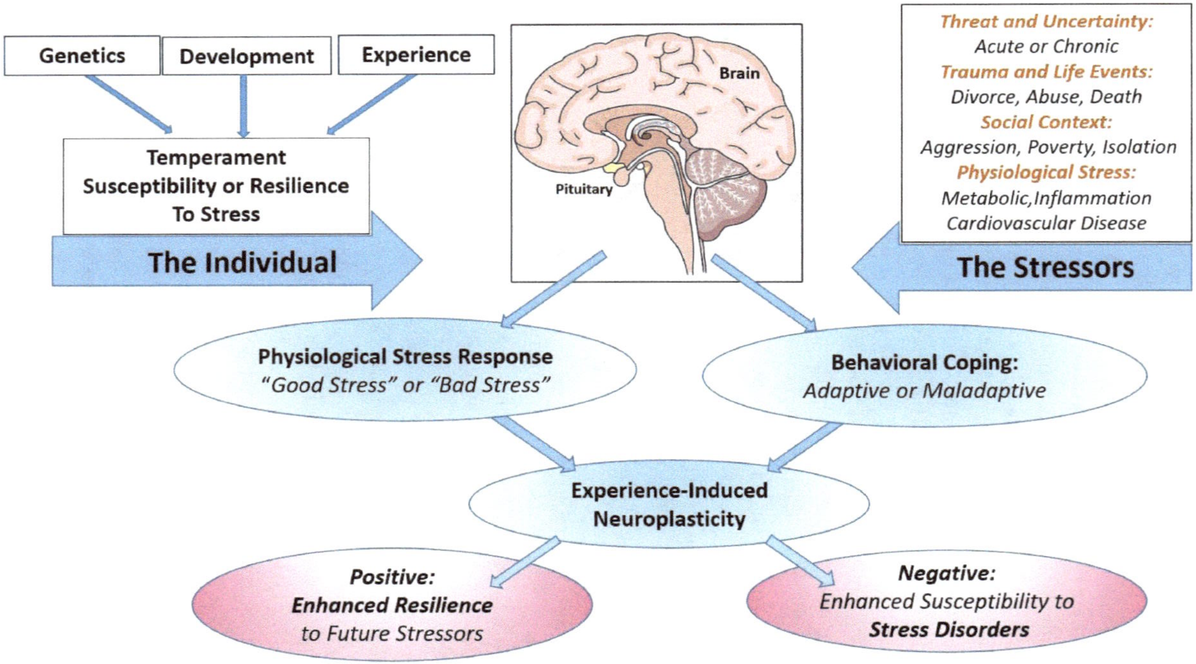

FIGURE 1-1 The interplay between the factors that contribute to an individual's susceptibility to stress and various stressors.
NOTE: The brain's ability to adapt and reorganize by forming new connections in response to lived experience (neuroplasticity) is mediated by physiological and behavioral responses and ultimately influence an individual's reaction to future stressors.
SOURCES: Presented by Huda Akil on March 24, 2025; adapted from McEwen and Akil.

often described as *allostatic load*, which refers to the wear and tear on the body caused by prolonged and repeated stress—can lead to physiological changes in the hippocampus and impair behavior, decision making, and judgment, pushing individuals into survival mode (see Figure 1-2).

To counteract these harmful effects, understanding the biology of resilience is important. Resilience is built through a dynamic interplay of growth factors and neuroplasticity that shapes how people handle stress from infancy through old age (Aurbach et al., 2015; Evans et al., 2004; Turner et al., 2012). However, resilience is not solely a biological process—it is also shaped by environmental and social factors. In a research study with college freshmen at the University of Michigan, Akil recalled that initially, genetic markers offered only a modest forecast of who might develop depression, but as the pandemic unfolded, the real differentiator was the perception of social support (Turner et al., 2023). She added that even those with low genetic risk were not immune when the comforting effects of genuine support faded. Akil reflected that this study revealed that there are multiple types of resilience, genetic and nongenetic, and that psychosocial factors such as social support matter.

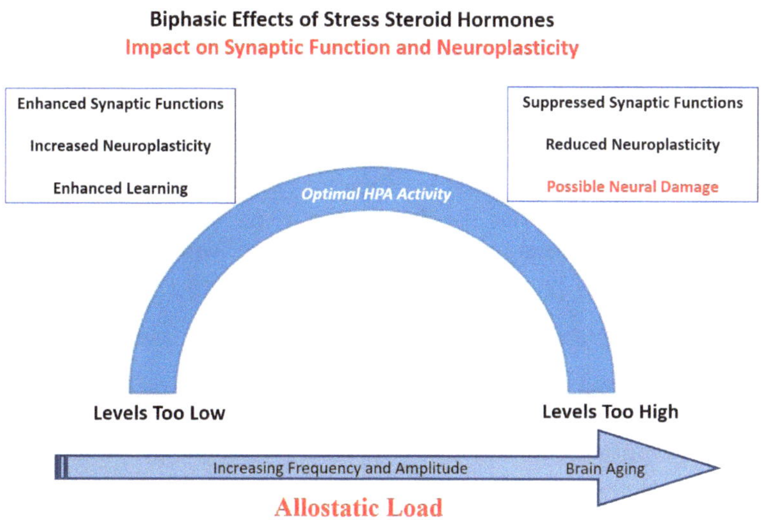

FIGURE 1-2 The biological effects of allostatic load.
NOTES: In response to stress, hormones like glucocorticoids and key signaling molecules serve a dual role. In balanced amounts, they help the brain adapt and learn. However, when these chemicals are produced in excess or in an imbalanced way, they can undermine resilience and even cause harm. When the natural ability to recover is compromised—as is often seen in mood disorders—additional support or treatment may be needed to restore balance.
SOURCES: Presented by Huda Akil on March 24, 2025; adapted from McEwen and Akil. ©2020. CC-BY 4.0.

Akil underscored the importance of preventing stress disorders, but prevention requires the ability to predict susceptibility and resilience in a given individual as a prelude to intervention. The Michigan Freshmen Study on Stress and Resilience showed that prediction is indeed possible (Turner et al., 2023). Akil coined the term "stress fitness" to define the essential process of building a healthy stress response, emphasizing that resilience can be trained and developed throughout life just like physical fitness—even in old age. By understanding and actively improving stress management, individuals can foster a healthier response to life's challenges.

WORKSHOP OBJECTIVES

The workshop aimed to address the rising prevalence of stress-related disorders and explore how resilience research can be strengthened through neurobiological insights (see Box 1). It included five sessions that spanned foundational topics such as the biological mechanisms of resilience and stress, as well as applied discussions on public health interventions and translational science. Personal resilience narratives from two individuals with stress-related disorders transformed abstract scientific discussions into tangible real-world insights.

In summary, this workshop provided a unique platform to advance scientific understanding and inspire new avenues for addressing the pressing challenges of stress and resilience. Emerging insights from research, such as the identification of biological markers of resilience and the benefits of perceived social support, underscored the potential for science to illuminate pathways toward fostering resilience in diverse populations, including children, adolescents, parents, and historically marginalized groups, and in varied contexts, including homes, communities, and workplaces.

ORGANIZATION OF PROCEEDINGS

This Proceedings of a Workshop is designed to summarize the discussions and presentations delivered throughout the workshop. Chapter 2 presents the narratives of two individuals who have demonstrated resilience in overcoming stress-related disorders, thereby grounding the discussion in authentic, real-world insights. Chapter 3 examines the neurobiological mechanisms of stress and resilience, setting a scientific foundation for the narrative. Chapter 4 then focuses on the importance of timing across the lifespan, while Chapter 5 explores other bodily manifestations of stress and resilience. Chapter 6 discusses clinical and public health interventions that translate these insights into actionable interventions, and Chapter 7 offers a comprehensive exploration of opportunities for promoting resilience. The references are provided in Appendix A and the workshop agenda in Appendix B.

BOX 1-1
Statement of Task

A planning committee of the National Academies of Sciences, Engineering, and Medicine will host a 1.5-day public workshop that brings together leaders and experts across sectors and disciplines (e.g., neuroscience, psychology, neurodevelopment, public health, medicine, and education) to explore the application of neurobiological insights on stress for building resilience.

Invited presentations and discussions may:

- Review scientific evidence on the global rise of stress, differences among populations, and the relationship between stress and development of systemic disorders (e.g., psychiatric, neurological, metabolic, cardiovascular, and autoimmune), highlighting specific examples.
- Examine recent discoveries illuminating the neurobiological mechanisms of stress susceptibility, distinct mechanisms of resilience, and individual differences in response to stress and building resilience.
- Consider the role of both childhood neurodevelopment and neuroplasticity across the lifespan in building early life and lifelong resilience (as opposed to stress susceptibility) and discuss effective approaches for optimizing resilience during critical and sensitive periods of neurodevelopment.
- Explore how these findings could inform public health programs and education to promote resilience to stress.
- Discuss research gaps and opportunities for studying resilience across research, clinical, and public settings.

A planning committee will develop the agenda for the workshop, select and invite speakers and discussants, and moderate the discussions. Following the workshop, proceedings of the presentations and discussions will be prepared by a designated rapporteur in accordance with institutional guidelines.

2

Lived-Experience Perspectives on Building Resilience

Highlights

- Resilience is not just an innate personal trait but a process developed through adversity. Building resilience requires conscious effort, support, and a willingness to reframe challenges as opportunities for growth. (Birto, Nelson)
- Stigma surrounding mental illness coupled with systemic failures within health care and government policy remain pervasive barriers to accessible and effective mental health treatment and recovery. (Birto, Nelson)
- Support systems and community connections are vital to recovery. Healing is not a solitary journey; whether through peer networks, mentorship, or advocacy, surrounding oneself with people who understand the experience of mental illness fosters resilience and encourages sustained progress. (Birto, Nelson)

NOTE: This list is the rapporteurs' summary of points made by the individual speakers identified, and the statements have not been endorsed or verified by the National Academies of Sciences, Engineering, and Medicine. They are not intended to reflect a consensus among workshop participants.

Huda Akil reflected on an earlier conversation with Indida Birto, who was a researcher at Emory University Rollins School of Public Health and a service plan coordinator at Here's to Life, Inc. at the time of the workshop. Birto shared with Akil her personal concept of resilience through the Japanese art of Kintsugi—where imperfections are embraced and transformed into strength (see Figure 2-1). "That is another way of looking at resilience," said Akil, emphasizing how lived experience can provide a different lens through which to examine resilience. This chapter explores the journeys of individuals who have built resilience through their lived experiences, enriched by a cultivated social support system and advancements in science.

A SPARK IN THE DARKNESS: ELECTRICITY AS MEDICINE

The journey of Jon Nelson—member of the board of directors of the American Brain Coalition, a lived-experience council of One Mind, a director of lived experience for Motif Neurotech, and Chief Pulverize Officer at Pulverize the Stigma—is a testament to the complexities of living with treatment-resistant major depressive disorder and the resilience that can emerge from the darkest moments. A self-described "serious mental illness lived-experience activist," Nelson has dedicated his life not only to overcoming his own struggles but also to voicing the challenges faced by countless individuals battling the relentless grip of depression.

In 2012 Nelson was diagnosed with major depressive disorder, a condition that swiftly escalated into a relentless treatment-resistant battle lasting nearly a decade. During those years, his only constant was a deep, pervasive desire to die—a sentiment he described with stark candor. Despite trying every available medical intervention, he found himself descending into what he plainly calls "hell." It was this despair that eventually drove him to participate in a clinical trial at Mount Sinai Hospital under the care of Helen Mayberg. The procedure required an intense, eight-hour neurosurgical intervention to install a device that delivers 22.5 million electrical pulses per day to his brain.

Almost immediately after the surgery, Nelson experienced what he calls a "bonus life." The profound change was "unmistakable," he noted: The constant suicidal ideation evaporated, and he found himself liberated from the disease that had long warped his perception of life. "Electricity is my medicine," he later reflected, underscoring the transformative impact of deep brain stimulation. Yet this newfound relief was coupled with an unforeseen challenge—the reawakening of genuine emotion. In the early days following his recovery, he relished small moments of normalcy—walking his dog, enjoying lunch with friends—but about six weeks postsurgery, the resurgence of familiar feelings of sadness, stress, and even anger forced him to confront a new reality. "I have to learn how to deal with sadness. I can now feel again," he recounted, highlighting the delicate task of relearning to navigate life's emotional spectrum.

This period of readjustment was not a solo journey. Nelson formed a community with four other individuals who, like him, had undergone the same procedure. Their quarterly Zoom meetings became a space for shared vulnerability, where fears of relapse lingered. Despite the collective relief of emerging from the clutches of treatment-resistant depression, each member carried an abiding anxiety—a stark reminder that the specter of their former condition was never fully gone. "If this comes back, I don't think I can survive," Nelson admitted, capturing the persistent tension between hope and fear.

Amid his personal struggles, Nelson did not shy away from confronting broader societal issues. His narrative highlighted the stigmatization faced by those with mental illness and how the needs and realities of these communities are often dismissed by health care and societal systems. He recalled the compassionate care he finally experienced at Mount Sinai Hospital—being "looked in the eye" and genuinely believed—against the backdrop of chronic neglect, the repeated insurance denials and societal indifference, that had unduly burdened him for years.

At the heart of Nelson's story lies a deeply personal definition of resilience. For him, resilience is not an abstract concept but the very act of facing each new day despite lingering fears and emotional challenges. "Resilience is waking

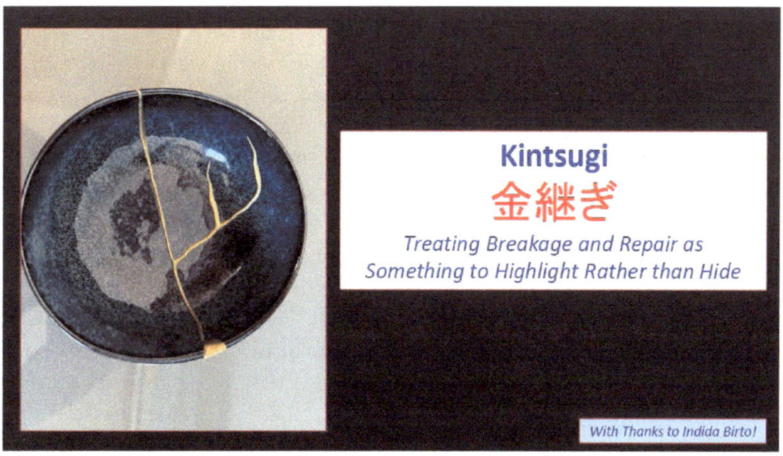

FIGURE 2-1 The Japanese art of Kintsugi.
NOTES: A concept, shared by Indida Birto, that highlights repair through casting gold on the fractures of pottery. This bowl, shared by Huda Akil, resembles a neuron and symbolizes the beauty of resilience. Its fractured areas are repaired with gold, representing strength and transformation.
SOURCE: Presented by Huda Akil on March 24, 2025.

up every single day," he asserted—a motto that frames his ongoing struggle. His resilience is expressed not only through his personal transformation but also in his commitment to forming peer support networks and pushing for change. Even as he battles uncertainties about medication adjustments and the possibility of relapse, his unwavering determination to transform anger into actionable advocacy stands as a powerful beacon for others.

His account is not solely about the marvels of biomedical intervention or the triumph of modern neurosurgery. It is, at its core, a candid exploration of the human spirit—a call to recognize that even in the face of overwhelming darkness, the act of simply rising each morning constitutes an extraordinary form of resilience.

MENDING LIFE'S FRACTURES WITH GOLDEN STRENGTH

Indida Birto shared her personal journey with resilience—a path defined not by innate strength but by the ongoing work of overcoming adversity. Drawing on her extensive background in recovery, HIV care, case management, and research, Birto's narrative weaves together a story of hardship and emerging purpose. Birto focused on the metaphor of Kintsugi (mentioned previously by Akil), explaining that when someone navigates life's challenges and mends the metaphorical cracks with gold, they become even more valuable (see Figure 2-1).

Birto's story begins with a candid reflection on her early years—a time marked by intergenerational family struggles. Growing up in an immigrant family burdened by substance use disorder and behavioral health challenges, she recalled a childhood shadowed by insurmountable difficulties and trapped by circumstances beyond her control. In an environment where understanding and support were limited, her early life set the stage for a gradual yet profound transformation.

A turning point in her narrative was the gradual reframing of adversity. Birto vividly recalled a period when every setback seemed difficult to overcome, yet over time, she began to reimagine her hardships as a service to others. In a resonant moment, she stated, "each of us is a testament to the miracle of resilience. You are a miracle." This declaration underscored a pivotal shift: understanding that the very experiences that once seemed to define her limitations were, in fact, the building blocks of a renewed self. By viewing each challenge as an opportunity for growth, Birto illustrated how the process of resilience involves continual adaptation and learning from each stumble along the way.

Central to her message is the importance of community and self-compassion. Throughout her journey, Birto embraced support systems ranging from crisis counselors to peer networks, emphasizing that even the smallest gestures of kindness can help neutralize negative experiences. She poignantly remarked, "Once you make the place upstairs [your mind] a safe place, your life will blossom." Her words evoke an image of inner space as a sanctuary, one that, when nurtured, allows for personal transformation. In this environment of self-kindness, even setbacks—likened to falling and hitting one's head repeatedly—can become the stepping stones toward building a resilient identity.

Birto's experiences also brought to light the fundamental role of small everyday moments in the pursuit of resilience. She recounted instances where, despite significant challenges, moments as simple as observing a worm on the ground or enjoying the beauty of a cherry blossom contributed to a sense of wonder and gratitude. These seemingly trivial details, woven into the fabric of her daily life, reminded her that resilience blooms not only from grand triumphs but also from the cumulative impact of minor, magical moments.

Her narrative, replete with both vulnerability and strength, offered a reflection on resilience as an ongoing journey rather than a fixed destination. In sharing her life's trajectory—from the depths of despair to experiences of small yet significant victories—Birto invited the workshop participants to recognize that every personal struggle, every setback, has the potential to contribute to a broader tapestry of growth and community connection.

3

Understanding the Neuroscience of Stress and Resilience

Highlights

- In stress-susceptible mice, suppressing the activity of the lateral septum—a brain region that regulates social behavior—reduces avoidance behavior and improves social engagement, pointing to its role in shaping stress-related information. (Russo)
- Neural population, fear extinction, and genetic studies indicate that the amygdala may play a large role in stress susceptibility and resilience. (Cameron, Kheirbek, Ressler)
- Both preclinical and human studies have shown sex differences in stress susceptibility and resilience, emphasizing the need to consider biological sex when designing resilience-building interventions or treatments. (Baratta, Cameron)
- The long-term effects of trauma and resilience can span generations, suggesting that reducing stress in parents may foster greater emotional stability and adaptability in future generations. (Ressler)
- Resilience is dynamic and can be influenced by many factors, such as early life experiences (e.g., maternal separation), behavioral control, physical activity, antidepressants, support systems, sleep quality, and household stability. (Baratta, Cameron, Kheirbek, Ressler, Russo)

- Inconsistent definitions of resilience across research fields make translational comparisons challenging. (Hyde)

NOTE: This list is the rapporteurs' summary of points made by the individual speakers identified, and the statements have not been endorsed or verified by the National Academies of Sciences, Engineering, and Medicine. They are not intended to reflect a consensus among workshop participants.

Michael Milham, senior child and adolescent psychiatrist, chief science officer, and founding director of the Center for the Developing Brain at the Child Mind Institute, described how the use of different preclinical (rodents, nonhuman primates) and clinical models has helped to uncover fundamental neural mechanisms of stress, examine how developmental and social factors shape responses, and ultimately provide insights into mental health across the lifespan. He emphasized that the findings from the speakers' research offer crucial insights for designing interventions that better support individuals and communities facing adversity.

THE ROLE OF THE LATERAL SEPTUM IN SOCIAL TRAUMA

Scott Russo, professor of neuroscience and director of the Center for Affective Neuroscience and the Brain-Body Research Center at the Icahn School of Medicine at Mount Sinai, introduced a series of studies that use rodent models to probe the neural impact of negative social experiences. He noted that social behavior, maintained by evolutionary pressures, has played a critical role in enabling animals to detect predators, allocate limited resources, and enhance reproductive success. Russo added that these interactions offer positive affective experiences and serve as natural rewards. Yet when social experiences become traumatic, he explained, the very networks that provide support may transform into sources of distress. More specifically, Russo detailed how the brain encodes negative social experiences through activation of the lateral septum, a brain region associated with regulating social behaviors (Li et al., 2023). This activation reportedly suppresses downstream reward pathways, such as those projecting from the nucleus accumbens, a brain region important in processing reward, positive reinforcement, and pleasure (Li et al., 2023). This suppression of the reward pathways ultimately leads to generalized social avoidance, and this effect is amplified by social trauma (Li et al., 2023). Therefore, Russo's team employed a chemogenetic[1] approach by using an inhibitory designer receptor exclusively activated by a designer drug (DREADD) to precisely silence lateral septum activity, which in turn reduced avoidance and boosted social interaction. Russo underscored two key brain-behavior features associated with traumatic social experiences: a blunted response to natural rewards (anhedonia) and an accentuated threat response during exposures to ambiguous stress signals (Li et al., 2023).

Russo also described a chronic social defeat stress model where genetically identical mice are subjected to brief five-minute bouts of social bullying from an aggressor mouse, repeated over a span of 10 days (Krishnan et al., 2007; Li et al., 2023; Navarrete et al., 2024). He demonstrated that, despite their uniform genetic background, experimental mice exhibit divergent responses: roughly half become stress susceptible while the other half show signs of resilience. Through modifications in standard paradigms (including resident intruder and social preference tests), his data suggested that stress not only triggers state-dependent neural activity but also leads to a generalized form of fear that impairs positive social interactions. Russo inferred that the lateral septum may be acting as a sensor that operates within the particular context of a stressful environment; the lateral septum registers environmental threat and also interacts dynamically with the brain's reward systems to shape behavior. Rather than simply reflecting an absence of interest in social stimuli, these data suggest, the lateral septum may inhibit the brain's capacity to experience social interactions as rewarding.

THE DYNAMICS OF THE AMYGDALA–HIPPOCAMPAL CIRCUIT IN STRESS RESILIENCE

Mazen Kheirbek, an associate professor in the Department of Psychiatry at the University of California, San Francisco, and a member of the Kavli Institute for Fundamental Neuroscience, extended the discussion by explaining how real-time monitoring of neural population dynamics could help predict different stress responses in a rodent model of chronic stress. Kheirbek's work harnesses Neuropixels[2] to obtain simultaneous live recordings of large populations of neurons within the amygdala and hippocampus. Analysis of a

[1] Chemogenetics is a method used in neuroscience that involves genetically engineering receptors to respond exclusively to synthetic chemical ligands. This allows researchers to precisely control cellular activity, particularly in neurons, by administering specific compounds that activate or inhibit these receptors without affecting natural signaling pathways (Menard and Russo, 2018).

[2] Neuropixels is a silicon digital neural probe that allows for large-scale neural recording

six-minute time period revealed that the neural activity in stress-susceptible mice shifted through a greater number of distinct population states in the amygdala compared to that of control and stress-resilient populations (Xia et al., 2025). This variation in amygdala signaling emerges precisely during decision-making moments—such as when choosing between water and sucrose solutions—thereby potentially interfering with the normal valuation of rewards (Xia et al., 2025). Kheirbek explained that these inherent differences in the spontaneous resting activity of these regions can distinguish between control, stress-resilient, and stress-susceptible mice (Xia et al., 2025).

A particularly striking observation was the increased synchrony of activity between the ventral hippocampus and the amygdala in stress-resilient mice immediately before high-reward decisions, said Kheirbek (Xia et al., 2025). The data revealed that in stress-resilient mice, the ventral hippocampus and amygdala become more synchronized immediately before making high-value reward choices (Xia et al., 2025). Leveraging this observation, Kheirbek's group used DREADD—the chemogenetic approach that employs designer receptors—to artificially enhance the correlation between these regions in stress-susceptible mice (Xia et al., 2025). By boosting this synchrony between the amygdala and hippocampus in stress-susceptible mice, Kheirbek's group was able to rescue disrupted reward processing and reduce anhedonia-related behaviors.

STRESS CONTROLLABILITY AND SEX DIFFERENCES IN NEURAL RESPONSES

Michael Baratta, an assistant professor of behavioral neuroscience at the University of Colorado Boulder, pivoted the discussion toward how the ability to physically control a stressor—a coping behavior called stressor controllability—can buffer the impacts of stress and build resilience. Because resilience is deeply rooted in neural processing, Baratta's research examines how stress-related experiences shape the rodent prefrontal cortex, basal ganglia, and limbic structures—key brain regions involved in decision making, emotional regulation, and adaptive behavior. His work focuses on how experiential factors like physical activity, stress coping, pharmacological resilience, and dominant status influence these neural circuits. He explained that human resilience is closely linked to coping strategies, which are categorized into emotion management and direct conflict resolution. While coping strategies are difficult to model in animals, behavioral control over stressors is a notable

with single-cell resolution. For more information, see https://www.neuropixels.org/ (accessed June 11, 2025).

exception and is commonly studied using an instrumental learning task. During the instrumental learning task, rats learn to turn a wheel to stop tail shocks (controllable stress), affecting both the rat itself and a yoked partner in the uncontrollable condition. For the uncontrollable stress subject, turning the wheel has no effect. Baratta explained that the physical stressor is the same between conditions, emphasizing that the experimental manipulation rests solely on the degree of control exercised over stopping the stressor. Baratta noted that decades of research have shown that when subjects are exposed to adverse events that they cannot control or escape, the stress can overwhelm certain brain pathways, leading to behavioral symptoms analogous to learned helplessness or depression (Maier and Watkins, 2005).

However, Baratta's data revealed a crucial sex difference: Behavioral control was not protective in female rats (Baratta et al., 2018). Female rats in the controllable stress condition displayed similar symptoms of learned helplessness and depression as both male and female counterparts in the uncontrollable stress condition. Further investigations revealed that male rats primarily relied on a goal-directed pathway through the dorsomedial striatum, where actions were driven by outcome-based decision making. In contrast, female rats with behavioral control primarily relied on a habit-based pathway through the dorsolateral striatum driven by reflexive and automatic decision making. Moreover, in female rats, excess dopamine release in the prefrontal cortex appeared to suppress the goal-directed system, thereby limiting the protective benefits of behavioral control (Baratta et al., 2018). These findings suggest that the equivalent expression of behavioral control can be governed by two very different neural circuit mechanisms in males and females, with major implications for understanding stress resilience across sexes, said Baratta. He underscored the importance of examining resilience-specific mechanisms—not just the mechanisms of uncontrollable stress—thereby offering a nuanced view of how sex differences may shape health outcomes in response to stress.

EARLY LIFE STRESS AND THE ROLE OF SOCIAL SUPPORT

Bridging animal models to human developmental studies, Judy Cameron, professor of psychiatry, neuroscience, obstetrics, gynecology, and behavioral and community health sciences at the University of Pittsburgh, provided important context on the timing of stress exposure. Drawing from her nonhuman primate studies, Cameron contrasted outcomes in infant monkeys experiencing maternal separation at different developmental stages. For example, monkeys separated at one month of age exhibited a persistent increase in social avoidance, whereas those separated as one-week-olds, although initially distressed, later demonstrated some recovery when provided with timely social support through the comfort of a foster mother. She found that all 200 genes she examined in the amygdala were changed in three-month-old monkeys that experience just one week of early maternal separation. She highlighted that the gene that changed the most in the one-week- and one-month-separated animals was the soluble guanylate cyclase gene, identifying it as part of the nitric oxide pathway in the amygdala. Additionally, Cameron described a strong correlation between guanylate cyclase expression levels and social behavior, with lower expression associated with increased social avoidance. Cameron's research also showed that even a few days' delay in providing an adoptive mother's support could result in markedly different long-term social behaviors (see Figure 3-1). She stressed that the timing of social support interventions in the immediate aftermath of early life stress is a critical factor for promoting resilience.

In parallel, her work with young children exposed to family stress underscored the mediating role of sleep in socioemotional and executive functioning.

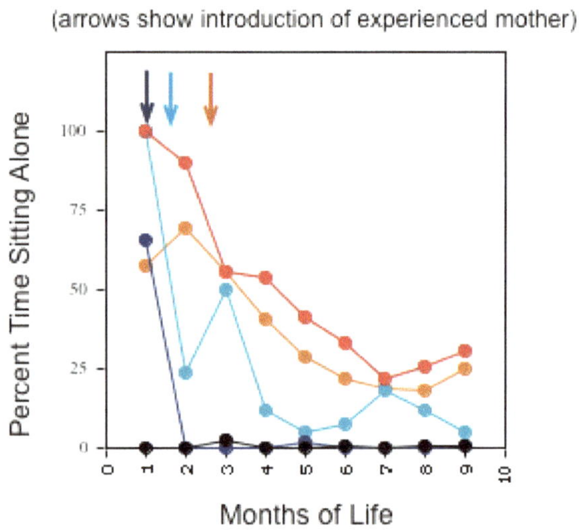

FIGURE 3-1 Earlier introduction of a foster mother "monkey" significantly enhances social recovery, helping the separated infant monkey reintegrate more effectively.
NOTES: Percentage of time infant monkeys spend sitting alone following one-week maternal separation. Social recovery is compared across different intervention points: foster mother introduced at 25 days (purple), 35 days (blue), and 45 days (orange) postseparation. Additionally, behavioral outcomes are contrasted with infant monkeys who received no foster mother (red) and those who never experienced maternal separation (black).
SOURCE: Presented by Judy Cameron on March 24, 2025.

Her research indicates that children exposed to low resources, poor caregiver education, and chronic family stress exhibited impairments in social-emotional skills, attention, and problem solving. Importantly, Cameron identified sleep as a significant mediator of these effects. In her studies, children growing up in adverse environments who nonetheless got sufficient, quality sleep were more likely to maintain better developmental outcomes, despite the stressors. She noted that in statistical models, sleep appears to buffer the detriments of stress on children's cognitive and social development. This finding points to sleep as a potential lever for resilience: Ensuring healthy sleep habits may help children cope with or recover from the effects of early adversity. During the discussion period, sleep was also raised as a protective factor to stressors.

Cameron also observed notable sex differences in how stress affects child development. For instance, in her data, exposure to high adversity was linked to increased attention problems in boys, whereas girls did not show the same degree of impact on attention (Cameron et al., 2017). This suggests that biological sex may influence vulnerability or resilience to certain stress-related outcomes, an important factor to consider when designing interventions, said Cameron. Factors like the timing of stress exposure, the availability of supportive relationships, and even basic health behaviors such as sleep may all shift a child's trajectory toward susceptibility to stress and resilience. With better understanding of these developmental mechanisms, early life interventions may be tailored to foster resilience in vulnerable children.

RECOVERY, PLASTICITY, AND INTERGENERATIONAL MECHANISMS OF RESILIENCE

Kerry Ressler, chief scientific officer at McLean Hospital and professor at Harvard Medical School, focused on understanding resilience through the lens of trauma recovery and the neurobiological mechanisms underlying adaptation after stress. Drawing from the Grady Trauma Project, a large-scale study of civilian trauma in an urban, historically marginalized African American population, Ressler highlighted the prevalence of post-traumatic stress disorder (PTSD) and depression, noting that resilience moderates these effects (Wingo et al., 2010; Wrenn et al., 2010). He explained how genetic factors contribute to stress vulnerability. Ressler cited recent Psychiatric Genomics Consortium findings that identified 95 loci (genetic locations) linked to PTSD risk (Nievergelt et al., 2024). Moreover, they found that variations in the corticotropin-releasing hormone receptor—an important regulator of stress response, mood, metabolism, and other physiological functions—play a key role in individual differences in PTSD susceptibility (Nievergelt et al., 2024).

Ressler highlighted fear extinction, the process by which repeated passive exposure to fear-related stimuli, without reinforcement, gradually weakens the fear response, as a model of resilience. His work began with an antibiotic drug (D-cycloserine) that enhances the brain's ability to adapt and form new connections (or neural plasticity) by influencing specialized proteins important in learning and memory, called N-methyl-D-aspartate receptors. Ressler explained that their early studies showed that D-cycloserine could accelerate fear extinction in anxiety disorders, PTSD, obsessive compulsive disorder, and social anxiety. However, later findings revealed that when memories are reactivated, D-cycloserine could inadvertently strengthen fear memories rather than inhibit them (Ressler et al., 2004; Walker et al., 2002). Ressler suggested that some clinical trials may have faltered because not everyone was engaging in effective fear extinction learning. He raised the question of whether neural plasticity is always beneficial or if it must be carefully directed to avoid unintended effects. He proposed that future research should focus on pinpointing specific cellular mechanisms that promote fear inhibition—rather than risk reinforcing fear memories. One promising direction comes from Andreas Lüthi's group, which identified "fear-off" neurons in the amygdala that activate specifically during extinction learning (Herry et al., 2008). Ressler emphasized the importance of understanding fear-off circuits in the amygdala to advance research on fear extinction and resilience.

He then connected this to intergenerational effects of trauma that demonstrated that children of mothers exposed to high levels of abuse face an increased physiological risk for stress-related responses (Jovanovic et al., 2011; Stenson et al., 2021). Ressler emphasized that this includes heightened startle reactions and increased sympathetic nervous system activation.

Building on this understanding of fear responses, Ressler discussed research on sensory modulation in the olfactory system. His lab found that mice conditioned to fear an odor developed enhanced neuronal and structural changes in the olfactory bulb, such as increased glomerular size (Jones et al., 2007). They also demonstrated that these changes were passed down to the next generation—even without direct exposure to the fearful odor (Dias and Ressler, 2014). Further research revealed that fear extinction reversed these structural changes, raising the question of whether resilience can be inherited (Morrison et al., 2015). Ressler referenced a study that found that when fathers underwent extinction training before mating, their offspring no longer exhibited fear-related structural changes (Aoued et al., 2019). Ressler suggested that treating the parental generation could break the cycle of fear transmission through behavioral and epigenetic mechanisms.

DISCUSSION

Translating from Animal Models to Human Interventions

Aleksandra Vicentic, a branch chief at the National Institute of Mental Health, opened by pointing out that while animal models offer clear insights into controlled factors like stress timing and context, translating these findings to the human experience is challenging. Milham challenged the panel to elaborate about how resilience and stress are defined across species, how findings can be translated between species, and the role of timing in these processes. Ressler explained that while basic science researchers often bear the responsibility for translating findings, psychiatry still struggles with achieving measurable, reproducible biomarkers and behavioral tests. He pointed out that psychiatric diagnoses have remained largely unchanged for a century, relying on self-reported feelings rather than objective markers. However, the shift toward biomarkers, quantitative behavioral approaches, and brain-based measures will improve reproducibility and facilitate translation across mammalian species. Cameron underscored the importance of treatment timing by noting that animal studies reveal limited time windows during which neural circuits remain malleable, suggesting that identifying similar windows in humans could improve treatment efficacy. "It isn't that one type of intervention at one time is always going to work," she added. Cameron noted that different stresses alter distinct circuits and advocated for precision in targeting interventions: "The science is telling us that we need to target our interventions to specific times and to specific stresses." Cameron also pointed out that while science supports early intervention, societal challenges make it difficult to reach children experiencing stress early.

Baratta emphasized the need for a framework that organizes behavioral and cognitive dimensions that contribute to resilience. He noted that different resilience factors—such as exercise, safety signals, and enhanced extinction learning—may operate through distinct pathways and mechanisms rather than affecting all aspects of resilience uniformly. Baratta also suggested that there must be a neural system that integrates these dimensions, allowing for behavioral flexibility and adaptation. He pointed out that freezing behaviors, for example, would limit one's ability to explore new contingencies, implying that resilience mechanisms need to be compatible with broader adaptive behaviors. Baratta also questioned whether there is a specific brain structure responsible for coordinating these interconnected resilience-promoting factors.

Adding a technological perspective, Kheirbek highlighted that advances like high-resolution functional magnetic resonance imaging and other direct neural recording techniques have emerged only in the past 10 to 20 years. These innovations in human research enable a reverse translation process, where observations in human studies guide further exploration in animal models. He concluded that this approach fosters a bidirectional integration between basic science and clinical research. Cameron supported the idea that moving between human and animal models can deepen understanding. She described how a chance meeting with Takao Hensch, a researcher from Boston Children's Hospital, led to a pivotal discovery—attention mechanisms observed in children mirrored findings from his studies in mice. This prompted Hensch to revisit his animal research, reconfirming this result. Cameron added that the mouse model provided a valuable opportunity to investigate neural mechanisms in greater detail, such as dopamine receptor changes in the anterior cingulate—insights that would have been impossible to examine directly in humans (Makino et al., 2024).

Brian Dias, an associate professor at the University of Southern California, asked how long-lasting the chemogenetic stimulation effects were and whether boosts were needed. Kheirbek stated that his team had not yet tested the long-term effects of chemogenetic stimulation, but they were actively investigating whether plasticity within the circuit could be induced to create lasting change. He referenced deep brain stimulation research, noting that repeated stimulation can enhance plasticity over time, leading to greater circuit excitability.

Luke Williamson Hyde, a professor of psychology at the University of Michigan, raised concerns about inconsistent definitions of resilience across research fields, making translational comparisons challenging. He explained that the National Institutes of Health convened researchers who had received funding via a specific grant-funding mechanism focused on resilience with projects ranging from child development to military veterans and PTSD. One goal of the meeting was to establish standardized definitions of resilience or standardized measures. However, after two days of discussion, they were unable to reach a consensus because resilience is highly context dependent. Hyde explained that different fields study resilience in distinct ways, making it difficult to apply a single definition across disciplines, but also that substantial work on resilience and its definitions in human developmental science has often not penetrated to researchers in other fields.

Demographic Factors Contributing to Resilience

A workshop participant asked Cameron whether her research, which identified sex differences, also examined ethnic, cultural, or racial differences in resilience and development. Additionally, the audience sought insight into trauma- and thriving-informed approaches to better distinguish resilience from depression, especially in diverse and vulnerable populations. Cameron explained that her studies, which included children from Canada and the

United States, have not found ethnic or racial differences despite examining diverse samples. She noted that this does not mean such differences do not exist, only that her team has not observed them. However, they did find sex differences, particularly in attention-related outcomes among males. She cautioned against assuming sex-based findings are absolute, suggesting that high levels of stress might impact girls in similar ways under certain conditions. Ressler added that in national cohort studies where racial or cultural differences have been observed in trauma or depression outcomes, those differences have almost always been moderated or mitigated by socioeconomic factors such as poverty, adversity, and access to green space. Kheirbek also acknowledged challenges in studying resilience at the population level, noting that resilient individuals are less likely to enroll in clinical trials because they are otherwise psychologically healthy. Ressler suggested the the ABCD (Adolescent Brain Cognitive Development) study as a valuable resource for examining resilience across healthy and at-risk populations, ensuring a broad symptom spectrum beyond strictly clinical samples.[3]

In a related line of inquiry, Herman Taylor, a cardiologist and director at the Cardiovascular Research Institute at Morehouse College of Medicine, asked whether experimental models account for acute-on-chronic adversity, where populations experience long-term generational hardship alongside new acute stressors, such as policy changes, violence, or environmental instability. He inquired whether any models exist to examine the vulnerability, susceptibility, and resilience associated with this compounded adversity. Ressler confirmed that models addressing acute-on-chronic adversity do exist, though the topic is complex and requires multifaceted approaches. He explained that in human studies, patterns of poverty and adversity tend to increase risk, particularly when a new trauma is added to childhood trauma, exacerbating susceptibility. Ressler added that in mouse models, researchers see similar effects: For example, mice exposed to chronic social defeat in adolescence display heightened fear responses and reduced ability to extinguish fear conditioning when tested in adulthood. He emphasized that the neural mechanisms underlying this process are complex, but there is clear evidence of an additive effect, where prior adversity amplifies the impact of later stressors.

The Dynamic Nature of Resilience

Vicentic posed a question on whether resilience is better understood as an innate trait or a flexible state that may be measured before or after trauma

[3] The ABCD study is a longitudinal study following the biological and behavioral development of children through adolescence and into adulthood. For more information, see https://abcdstudy.org/ (accessed June 11, 2025).

exposure. Building on that, she wondered if resilience exists as a trait prior to experiencing adversity or if it is instead a more positive coping strategy after adversity happens. In response, Ressler clarified that resilience is not merely the absence of vulnerability but rather the ability to bounce back or recover from adversity. He noted that neural circuit mechanisms may influence susceptibility or resilience differently as well. Ressler also brought forth the concept of "traumatic growth"—the idea that exposure to manageable levels of stress could, under the right conditions, catalyze personal development and better coping mechanisms. Beyond self-report measures, emerging techniques in the integration of machine learning with neuroimaging and behavioral studies may offer innovative ways to quantify these phenomena, although the conversation acknowledged that much work remains to capture the full continuum of resilience in diverse populations. Kheirbek pointed to animal model research, explaining that resilient mice exhibit unique neural activity compared to both unstressed controls and susceptible mice. He cited findings from Eric Nestler's lab, showing that dopamine neuron activity in the ventral tegmental area adapts uniquely in resilient mice and can be manipulated to promote behavioral resilience.

Indida Birto asked whether there is a predictable threshold for adverse childhood experiences (ACEs)—a "make-it-or-break-it" number—beyond which resilience becomes harder to maintain. She acknowledged that recovery is always possible but wondered whether a specific number of ACEs allows researchers to predict long-term outcomes. Cameron emphasized that adversity is often repeated throughout life, and early exposure increases the likelihood of experiencing additional adversity later. She pointed out that brain circuits develop until age 25, meaning that the timing, type, and affected neural circuits play a role in how adversity influences outcomes. Cameron concluded that there is no universal threshold, as each experience interacts uniquely with development. Ressler reinforced this by noting that PTSD rarely develops from a single trauma—instead, risk tends to increase with repeated interpersonal adversity. He added that much of childhood trauma is relational, such as ongoing abuse, which compounds over time. Ressler also highlighted a gap in self-reported trauma data, explaining that declarative memories form around ages three to four, while emotional memories begin at birth. This raised concerns that early adversity may impact individuals in ways that they cannot consciously recall, leading to underreported trauma histories in studies.

Factors That Can Foster Resilience

Another topic that generated considerable interest was whether positive enrichment following a stressor might push neural circuits toward a more resilient state. Frances Jensen, a professor of neurology and the chair of the neurology department at the Perelman School of Medicine at University of Pennsylvania, asked whether resilience could be actively fostered through enrichment rather than simply removing stressors. She wondered if introducing positive rewards at key moments—particularly in susceptible animals—could counteract stress-induced network dysfunction and promote lasting resilience. Cameron agreed that enrichment can be effective when applied while neural circuits remain plastic. She pointed out that stress affects multiple circuits over time, raising the question of whether targeted enrichment could influence different circuits at different developmental stages. Kheirbek highlighted research showing that enrichment can boost adult neurogenesis in the hippocampus, citing work by Chris Anacker and Rene Hen demonstrating its role in promoting resilience. Russo emphasized that environmental enrichment, physical activity, antidepressants, and social buffering all contribute to resilience in animal models. Baratta added that behavioral control during late adolescence in rats leads to longer-lasting protective effects compared to adulthood, suggesting critical windows where interventions may be more effective.

Alexa Ryan, a senior at Howard University at the time, asked whether certain stressors can increase resilience rather than decrease it. Ressler noted that there is a body of literature on traumatic growth, but much remains unclear. He suggested that controllability plays a key role, explaining that individuals who face stressors but have strong support systems—such as parents, mentors, or coaches—may develop a resilient, perseverant personality rather than experiencing learned helplessness. However, he acknowledged that more studies are needed to fully understand this process. Baratta reinforced that resilience emerges within adversity, explaining that resilience-related neural circuits require activation under stressful conditions to be protective. He emphasized that certain early life stressors can produce long-lasting resilience, but only if tied to adversity itself rather than occurring in a neutral setting. Ressler added a follow-up, referencing Tallie Baram's research on predictability despite negative experiences. He shared a powerful finding from his team's work at the Grady Trauma Project, where asking participants whether they grew up in a stable or unstable household proved to be a highly predictive factor for resilience outcomes, suggesting that stability—regardless of adversity—plays a crucial role in fostering resilience.

The Negative Effects of Sustained Resilience

Laura Bustamante, a postdoctoral researcher at Washington University in St. Louis, referenced the John Henryism hypothesis, which suggests that effortful active coping can be beneficial for those in advantaged positions (e.g., higher education) but can lead to negative health outcomes, such as cardiovascular issues, for individuals in disadvantaged circumstances. Bustamante wondered whether animal models could be used to explore these neurobiological interactions between resilient and vulnerable subjects. Russo agreed that resilience research raises important concerns, including for type-A individuals (individuals who tend to be perceived as highly motivated, goal-oriented, and independent) who exhibit high psychological resilience but increased cardiovascular risk. He explained that in their psychosocial stress models, mice that are susceptible to stress tend to show broad vulnerability across multiple domains, whereas resilient mice experience benefits beyond psychological adaptation, including lower cardiovascular disease risk and improved response to statins. However, he cautioned that this does not apply to all definitions of resilience. Baratta described his team's coping-with-stress paradigm, in which animals can turn a wheel to mitigate stress exposure, leading to long-term behavioral protection. However, he noted that while behavioral resilience improves, immune system activity, autonomic nervous system function, and endocrine responses remain elevated, suggesting that even resilient individuals may still experience physiological strain.

Digital Technologies and Biological Measurements

Milham asked about advancing behavioral measurement, particularly in relation to digital technologies. He sought insights into whether these tools could improve cross-species research and help integrate findings across the lifespan. Russo highlighted several digital tools that are expanding behavioral measurement capabilities, including smartphones, wearable devices, and natural language processing. He pointed out that smartphones can provide both active and passive data, such as texting patterns and behavioral insights, while wearable devices can measure physiological factors like heart rate, temperature, and sleep patterns. Russo emphasized that quantitative sleep tracking has improved significantly, allowing researchers to study sleep behaviors across mammals and apply findings to younger populations. He suggested that these technologies could play a crucial role in bridging behavioral research across species and the lifespan, offering new opportunities for data collection and analysis.

Eva Feldman, a neurologist at the University of Michigan, asked whether researchers are using the All of Us cohort[4] for their work and whether doing so would be valuable. She also inquired about the use of AI to integrate human data with preclinical findings. Cameron stated that her team is not using the All of Us cohort but is actively employing machine learning to analyze videotaped behavior in children and monkeys. She explained that

[4] All of Us is a National Institutes of Health program created to build a diverse database that can inform thousands of studies on a variety of health conditions. See https://allofus.nih.gov/article/program-overview (accessed June 11, 2025).

researchers are trained to observe specific behaviors, and AI could help identify overlooked behavioral patterns in developmental studies. Cameron noted that machine learning has already yielded valuable insights in rodent research. Ressler described All of Us as an exciting and large-scale initiative, though its data availability is still rolling out. He compared it to the ABCD cohort, which has been instrumental in developmental research, and predicted that All of Us will soon have a similar impact. Ressler also discussed AI applications, noting that researchers have used machine-learning tools like DeepLabCut for video-based behavioral analysis. While AI has been useful for genetic comparisons between animal models and humans, he acknowledged that researchers have yet to fully bridge the gap at the behavioral circuit level.

Sleep and Stress Management: Public Health and Cultural Perspectives

Diane Bovenkamp, vice president of scientific affairs at BrightFocus® Foundation, asked about leveraging population health approaches to improve sleep and stress management, particularly in public schools or health care settings. She suggested offering digital tools, such as apps like Calm, to support better sleep habits, noting that stressors like social media are often unpredictable. She also wondered whether a billing code for sleep interventions could encourage doctors and pediatricians to integrate preventive measures into routine care. Cameron emphasized that sleep plays a critical role in childhood development, serving as a mediator for cognitive, emotional, and problem-solving abilities. She noted that her team has studied sleep insufficiency and poor sleep quality, finding that 79 percent of children in their research do not get enough sleep. She acknowledged the potential for broad interventions but expressed caution about mass-scale programs without careful tailoring. Ressler expanded on intervention strategies, highlighting that short-term treatments like cognitive behavioral therapy and dialectical behavior therapy are effective in improving emotion regulation and cognitive flexibility. He suggested that integrating these interventions into school health programs or prenatal care could have wide-reaching benefits for resilience and mental health.

A workshop participant asked how sleep physiology, alongside factors such as emotional regulation, neuroendocrine function, and developmental timing, influences neural circuit vulnerability or protection against substance misuse, personal violence, and social defeat. The participant also inquired about whether sleep deprivation acts as a confounder, distorting study results by making it appear as though one factor causes another when, in reality, an unaccounted-for third variable is driving the relationship. Cynthia Rogers, the Blanche F. Ittleson Professor of Psychiatry and Pediatrics and vice chair and division director of Child and Adolescent Psychiatry at Washington

University in St. Louis, shared that her team, including Caroline Hoyniak, is studying maternal and child sleep through polysomnography and at-home sleep studies. She highlighted research showing that maternal sleep affects brain development, suggesting that child sleep is likely to play a significant role as well. While she acknowledged the clinical importance of sleep for development and mental health, she noted that her team has not yet examined sleep at the molecular or biological level. Catherine Jensen Peña, an assistant professor at the Princeton Neuroscience Institute, emphasized that disrupted sleep is a strong cross-species factor, making it a critical target for research in understanding neurodevelopmental effects. Nadine Burke Harris, senior advisor for the ACE Resource Network and former surgeon general of California, pointed out that sleep regulation affects the sympathoadrenal medullary and hypothalamic–pituitary–adrenal axes, which play key roles in stress and neuroendocrine function.

Dias asked Cameron about sleep education programs, specifically how cultural perspectives, such as co-sleeping, influence approaches to sleep education. He shared a personal experience of being shamed in parental groups for allowing co-sleeping, despite its prevalence globally. Cameron responded that her research on sleep education programs focuses primarily on families in impoverished conditions, where co-sleeping and frequent relocation are common. She explained that her team adapts sleep strategies to fit these realities, such as recommending that children sleep on portable mattresses in consistent locations to maintain a sense of stability. Cameron also described her approach to tailoring sleep routines, emphasizing practical strategies like having children wear the same T-shirt to sleep instead of conventional pajamas, which may be unrealistic for families in poverty. She underscored the challenges of external disruptions, such as violence and loud noises, and highlighted efforts to help parents manage these stressors to support their child's sleep.

In sum, preclinical research has focused on identifying the brain regions that underlie stress susceptibility and resilience, including the lateral septum, amygdala, dorsolateral striatum, and dorsomedial striatum. This can create opportunities for new targeted biomarkers, diagnostics, and treatments to cultivate resilience. However, there remains more to learn about the individual variability and dynamic nature of resilience, such as the contribution of factors such as sex, race, or cultural difference.

4

Critical and Sensitive Periods to Build Resilience

Highlights

- The timing of stress exposure determines which neural circuits are affected. Understanding these temporal dynamics allows researchers to design targeted interventions that align with specific developmental stages to optimize resilience-building. (Hyde, Meaney, Peña)
- An individual's environment shapes biological susceptibility to both stress and resilience. Understanding the mechanisms underlying responses to negative environmental factors—evident in both rodent and human studies—can be leveraged to develop interventions that buffer the long-term effects of severe stress and foster resilience. (Dias, Meaney, Peña, Rogers)
- Early life adversity alters key epigenetic markers, shaping neural circuits that regulate emotional and cognitive responses, that can persist into adulthood and amplify susceptibility to mental health disorders but also enhance responsiveness to environmental or neurobiological interventions. (Meaney, Peña)
- Parenthood induces neuroplastic changes that enhance caregiving and resilience but also increase vulnerability to mood disorders, reinforcing the need for targeted interventions during this life stage. (Saxbe)

- Many resilience factors do not operate as expected in contexts of extreme disadvantage, highlighting the need to address systemic barriers—like housing stability, food security, and access to education—alongside individual or parenting interventions. (Rogers)

NOTE: This list is the rapporteurs' summary of points made by the individual speakers identified, and the statements have not been endorsed or verified by the National Academies of Sciences, Engineering, and Medicine. They are not intended to reflect a consensus among workshop participants.

Brian Dias highlighted that critical periods are not solely times when stress profoundly impacts biological systems but also moments when resilience may be actively built. Dias emphasized that while infancy and adolescence are traditionally recognized as epochs where stress "gets under the skin," these periods also represent windows in which environmental inputs can promote adaptive responses (Taylor et al., 2025). The research presented in this chapter highlights how windows of heightened susceptibility to stress can also serve as periods when resilience may be built. As several workshop speakers described, the developmental trajectories—in utero, early childhood, adolescence, or the transition to parenthood—reflect an intricate dialogue between environmental challenges and biological adaptations (Ho and King, 2021).

ANIMAL MODELS OF EARLY LIFE STRESS AND EPIGENETIC PRIMING

Catherine Jensen Peña described work in rodent models that examines the interplay between early life stress and later vulnerability to the development of stress-related disorders. Peña's research utilizes paradigms of early stress across the lifespan (Peña, 2025; Peña et al., 2017, 2019). She noted that the timing of stress exposure in animal models should be selected with consideration of how it maps onto key periods of human brain development. In her own research, Peña's lab uses early life stress from postnatal days 10 to 17 in rodents, which she noted roughly corresponds to early childhood in humans for certain brain regions (Peña, 2025). These paradigms include a combination of early life stress such as maternal separation and resource restriction in rodents to mimic aspects of childhood adversity and adult stress, such as the chronic social defeat model shared earlier by Scott Russo. These manipulations, when combined, not only elevate risks for mood and anxiety disorders in animals but also create measurable changes in brain development long before stress symptoms emerge. Peña found that early life stress changes the expression of a number of genes across different brain regions related to nervous system development that last into adulthood. Furthermore, individuals with early life stress experiences that are exposed to stress as adults have epigenome-modulated changes in gene expression—that is, those life experiences influence gene activity without altering the underlying DNA sequence.

A key focus of Peña's investigation is epigenome priming. Epigenome priming refers to the process by which early life experiences—such as stress or environmental factors—modify chromatin structure, making specific regions of the genome more accessible for future transcriptional activation (Peña, 2025; Peña et al., 2017). This means that certain genes become "prepped" to respond more strongly to later stressors, shaping susceptibility to stress or resilience across development. She explained that early life stress is associated with persistent chromatin modifications—most notably monomethylation of histone 3 at lysine 4 (H3K4me1)—in brain areas important for reward and stress regulation, such as the ventral tegmental area and nucleus accumbens (Geiger et al., 2025). These epigenetic marks reduce the stress response threshold, triggering transcriptional change and therefore making the brain more sensitive to stress over time. Peña further discussed experiments where increased levels of the enzyme responsible for establishing these modifications, when experimentally overexpressed, led to elevated stress responsiveness at transcriptional, physiological, and behavioral levels (Peña, 2025; Peña et al., 2017, 2019). Moreover, her group explored thyroid hormone modulation as an upstream factor that may influence this epigenetic priming process, noting that early life stress could suppress active thyroid hormone levels, with brief synthetic thyroid hormone treatments in rodents later promoting resilience in the face of additional stress (Bennett et al., 2024).

ENVIRONMENTAL ENRICHMENT AS A PATHWAY TO RESILIENCE ACTIVATION

Michael Meaney, professor and James McGill Chair Emeritus in Medicine at McGill University, highlighted how both biological predispositions and environmental interventions can work together to promote resilience in individuals facing adversity. Meaney used a conceptual model for understanding the origins of psychopathology of stress and resilience called the stress diathesis framework. This framework suggests that under mild or positive environmental conditions, variations in mental health and well-being remain relatively small. However, as adversity increases, individual differences emerge—some people remain resilient, while others become more vulnerable to mental health challenges.

Meaney tested the stress diathesis framework using a rodent population exposed to environmental enrichment as a resilience model. He described how under conditions of sustained environmental enrichment during post-weaning to early adulthood, rodents display reduced stress reactivity and improved recovery after stressful events. Meaney's team has shown that enrichment not only increases neurogenesis in both dorsal and ventral regions of the hippocampus but also appears to boost executive functions like attention and cognitive flexibility (Pataskar et al., 2016; Zhang et al., 2018). This suggests that enrichment strengthens the brain's ability to adapt to stress.

A noteworthy aspect of Meaney's research was the translation of these findings to human populations. His team mapped the human orthologs—biological counterparts—of the genes upregulated in enriched mice and identified expression-based single nucleotide polymorphisms, which are DNA variations that functionally regulate gene expression. By compiling these variations into a targeted genetic profile, Meaney's team created a polygenic score for enrichment, reflecting the genetic capacity for the expression of enrichment-associated genes in humans. This score was then tested using data from more than 500,000 individuals through the UK Biobank,[1] providing insights into how individual genetic predispositions might shape resilience to stress and adversity. His team found that among individuals experiencing high levels of stress, those with higher enrichment polygenic scores exhibited fewer symptoms of depression and a lower probability of mood disorders. Importantly, this genetic influence was only observed in those exposed to substantial adversity—for individuals with low or modest stress levels, the polygenic score had no effect on depression symptoms. This suggests that enrichment-related gene expression functions as a buffer specifically when faced with significant life challenges.

Meaney discussed environmental enrichment as one potential approach to promoting resilience, showing that structured interventions—like classroom-based executive function training—may help enhance cognitive flexibility and emotional regulation, particularly in high-risk populations. He emphasized that resilience-building strategies should target both individual traits and broader structural factors, ensuring that families and communities have the stability needed to support positive developmental outcomes.

---

[1] For more information on the UK Biobank, see https://www.ukbiobank.ac.uk/ (accessed June 2, 2025).

PRENATAL AND EARLY CHILDHOOD ENVIRONMENTAL INFLUENCES ON BRAIN STRUCTURE

Cynthia Rogers focused on how social determinants of health impact infant brain development and early childhood social and emotional growth (Rakers et al., 2017). Her study, eLABE (Early Life Adversity, Biological Embedding, and Risk for Developmental Precursors of Mental Disorders), followed nearly 400 pregnant individuals through the third trimester and assessed how prenatal stress, inflammation, and environmental factors shaped neonatal brain structure (see Figure 4-1).

Rogers's findings showed that higher social disadvantage correlated with reduced neonatal brain volumes across multiple tissue types, affecting limbic structures like the amygdala and hippocampus. Structural connectivity in key white matter tracts that connect brain regions involved in emotion regulation, memory, and cognitive processing—such as the cingulum, fornix, and uncinate—was disrupted in infants exposed to greater prenatal social adversity. She identified maternal IL-6 levels (interleukin 6, a pro-inflammatory cytokine) as biological mediators, linking social disadvantage to altered neonatal brain volume (Sanders et al., 2024). Additionally, maternal sleep disturbances during pregnancy were associated with reductions in cortical volume and surface area at birth.

Rogers's research also explored environmental stressors like violent crime exposure (Brady et al., 2022). She found that even after adjusting for socioeconomic status and other environmental stressors, prenatal exposure to violent crime still had measurable effects on neonatal brain connectivity—particularly in regions like the amygdala and hippocampus. According to Rogers, this suggests that violent crime itself is a distinct factor influencing early brain development, beyond the broader effects of poverty or social disadvantage.

Turning to mechanisms that support resilience, Rogers's research found that supportive parenting plays a crucial role in early childhood development, particularly in cognitive and language growth (Leverett et al., 2025). While supportive parenting behaviors such as sensitivity and positive regard were associated with higher cognitive and language scores in children with moderate social disadvantage, they did not significantly improve outcomes for children with severe social disadvantage (Leverett et al., 2025). Therefore, Rogers observed that while supportive parenting can help buffer stress and promote development, it may not be enough on its own to offset the impact of extreme socioeconomic hardship.

Rogers also examined the Thrive Factor, a set of postnatal resilience supports—including nutrition, neighborhood safety, child sleep, positive caregiving, and environmental stimulation—to determine whether it could mitigate the effects of early social disadvantage on socioemotional function-

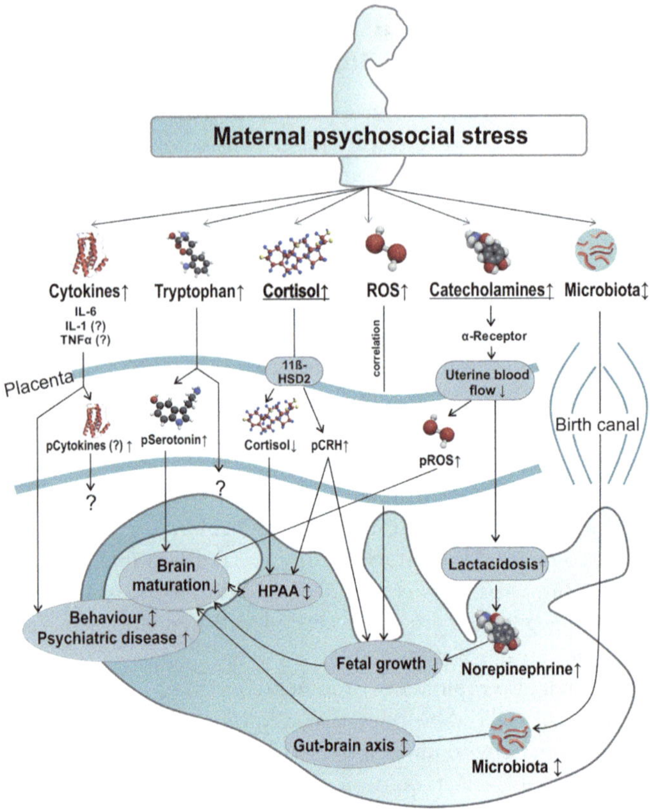

FIGURE 4-1 Maternal–fetal stress transfer occurs through multiple interconnected mechanisms that work synergistically to influence fetal development.
NOTES: Six potential mediators of maternal–fetal stress: cytokines, serotonin/tryptophan, cortisol, reactive oxygen species (ROS), catecholamines, and maternal microbiota. IL-6 = interleukin 6; IL-1 = interleukin 1; TNFα = tumor necrosis factor-alpha; p = phosphorylated; pCRH = phosphorylated corticotropin-releasing hormone; pROS = phosphorylated reactive oxygen species; HPAA = hypothalamic–pituitary–adrenal axis; α-receptor = alpha-adrenergic receptor; 11β-HSD2 = 11-beta-hydroxysteroid dehydrogenase type 2.
SOURCES: Presented by Cynthia Rogers on March 25, 2025; adapted from Rakers et al., 2017, and reproduced with permission from Elsevier.

ing, cognitive, and structural brain outcomes (Luby et al., 2024). Her findings revealed a complex relationship between these protective factors and socioeconomic status. Higher Thrive Factor scores were also associated with lower internalizing scores for children facing high levels of social disadvantage. While children from less disadvantaged backgrounds showed stronger cognitive and language benefits when exposed to high levels of Thrive Factor supports, children with more extreme social disadvantage did not experience the protective effects. She noted that for families facing greater social disadvantage, these protective influences were less effective at offsetting developmental disparities. Rogers emphasized that broader structural interventions, such as housing stability, access to health care, and community support, may be necessary to fully unlock the benefits of resilience support for children in highly disadvantaged environments. As her study enters its next phase, Rogers aims to further investigate child-level and community-based resilience mechanisms, including school and neighborhood supports that may shape long-term developmental outcomes.

EARLY CHILDHOOD ENVIRONMENTAL INFLUENCES ON ADOLESCENT BRAIN

Luke Williamson Hyde described how early adversity and neighborhood disadvantage affect brain development and behavior in children. He emphasized the significant role environmental influences play in shaping long-term outcomes. Hyde's work integrates longitudinal studies, neuroimaging, and behavior genetics to understand risk and resilience in youth growing up in high-stress environments.

Complementing Rogers's work, Hyde examined the effects of neighborhood violence on neural development in adolescents. Using functional magnetic resonance imaging (fMRI), his team found that youth exposed to higher community violence in early childhood exhibited increased amygdala reactivity to emotional stimuli, suggesting heightened sensitivity to threat (Gard et al., 2017, 2022a) and lower activity in the inferior frontal gyrus during inhibition and lower inhibitory control (Westerman et al., 2024) and greater activity in the ventral striatum, potentially increasing vulnerability to later mental health challenges. His work also highlighted how parenting serves as a stress buffer—youth with more nurturing caregivers showed less pronounced neural alterations, suggesting a buffering effect against adversity.

Consistent with earlier workshop discussions, the findings underscore that the effects of adverse exposures hinge on their timing. Early exposures, such as harsh parenting at age three or neighborhood disadvantage in early childhood, were linked to heightened amygdala activity—a subcortical region that develops early, which plays a key role in threat detection, emotional processing, and other functions (Gard et al., 2022b). And exposures later in development, including changes in parenting over childhood or neighborhood disadvantage during adolescence, relate to altered activity in the dorsal anterior cingulate cortex, a later-developing prefrontal area critical for emotion regulation (Hyde et al., 2022).

Broader adversities are inevitably funneled through immediate family experiences—a concept that is illustrated in Rand Conger's family stress model (Conger et al., 1992). In this model, poverty and economic pressure elevate parental stress, which then manifests as harsher parenting practices, ultimately linking to child mental health challenges. Hyde's brain data align with this view, reinforcing the idea that the impact of widespread adversity is mediated by more intimate, proximal interpersonal experiences that directly affect developmental outcomes.

In exploring the link between low-income neighborhoods and brain development, research has identified community violence as a key mechanism, with increased exposure predicting heightened amygdala responses to threat and altered ventral striatum activity to reward (Suarez et al., 2024; Westerman et al., 2024). However, positive social buffers emerge across multiple studies: Warm, involved parents both reduce the likelihood of exposure to such violence and temper its neurotoxic impact, while neighbors with strong protective norms further shield youth from these adverse effects (Gard et al., 2022a; Suarez et al., 2022). His findings emphasize the need for community-level interventions, advocating for policies that support families and reduce structural inequalities to encourage healthier brain development in children.

TRANSITION TO PARENTHOOD: A UNIQUE WINDOW FOR NEUROPLASTICITY

Darby Saxbe, a professor of psychology at the University of Southern California, examined the transition to parenthood as another critical window during which profound neuroplastic changes occur. Saxbe's research documents that the transition to parenthood is accompanied by large-scale brain remodeling, including reductions in gray matter volume in cortical regions involved in social cognition and mentalizing. Current research indicates that in mothers, such structural changes may represent an adaptive streamlining of neural circuits to facilitate efficient processing of infant cues (Carmona, 2024; Hoekzema et al., 2017).

Saxbe's work extends these observations to fathers, showing that men too exhibit changes—albeit subtler—in brain regions pertinent to caregiving and reward (see Figure 4-2). In fathers, greater reductions in cortical volume have been associated with stronger bonding to their infants and increased reports of parenting enjoyment (Martinez-Garcia et al., 2023). However, these neu-

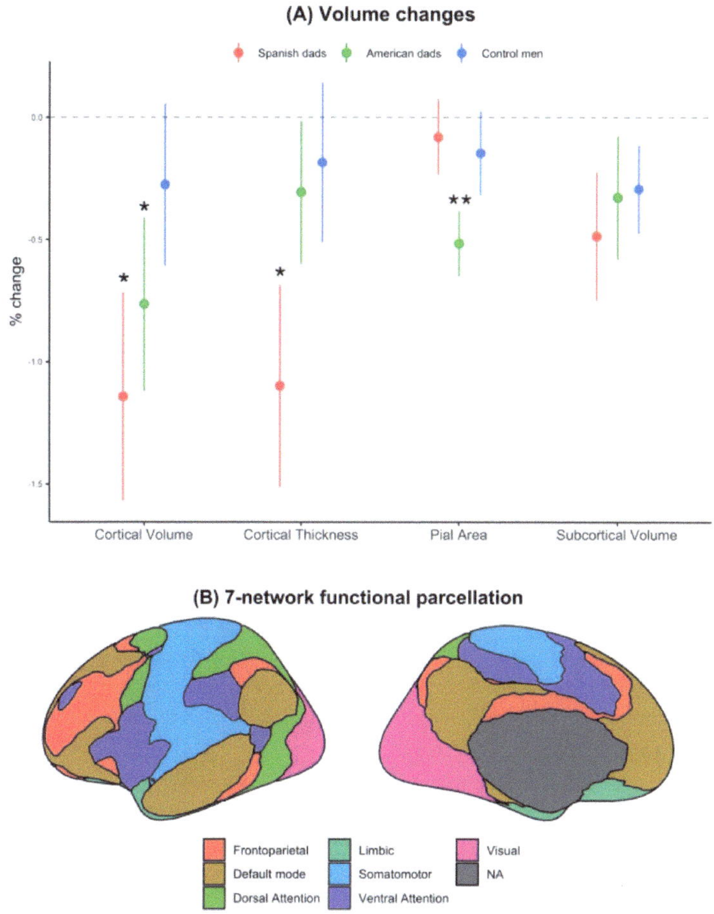

FIGURE 4-2 Paternal brain volume reduction during early fatherhood.
NOTES: Percentage of brain volume changes across different groups—Spanish fathers and Californian first-time fathers, and childless men. Statistical analysis using one-sample t-tests was performed to compare the percentage change in brain measures between prenatal and postnatal MRI scans. (A) shows the percentage of volume change for each brain measure. (B) presents a map of seven distinct functional networks in the brain, originally identified by Yeo and colleagues (2011), which highlight different brain regions involved in various cognitive and sensory functions. (C) displays the percentage of volume change within these seven functional networks.
SOURCES: Presented by Darby Saxbe on March 25, 2025; adapted from Martinez-Garcia et al., 2023. Reprinted by permission of Oxford University Press.

continued

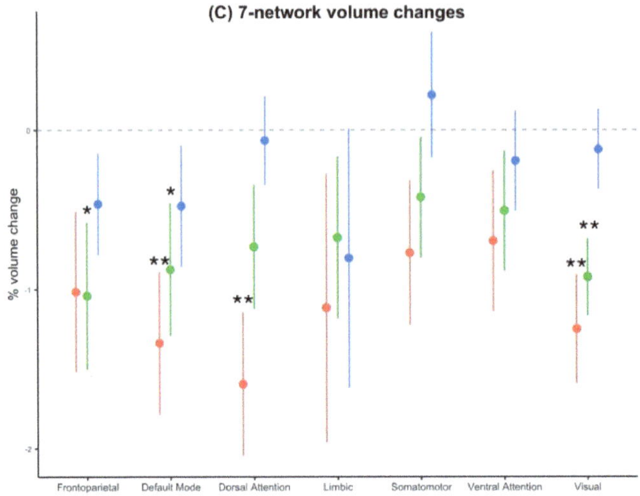

FIGURE 4-2 Continued.

robiological shifts were also linked to factors such as poorer sleep quality and heightened psychological distress, thus highlighting the dual nature of this window of plasticity: It may prime individuals for enriched caregiving while concurrently increasing susceptibility to mood disturbances if the environmental stress is high.

Moreover, emerging findings from Saxbe's laboratory indicate differential trajectories within specific regions, such as increases in hippocampal volume related to better caregiving outcomes (Saxbe and Martinez-Garcia, 2024). This evidence suggests that even within the overall pattern of remodeling observed during the transition to parenthood, individual differences may reflect compensatory mechanisms engaged to optimize parental functioning.

Saxbe also shared findings from her research team, led by Sofia Cardenas, on brain structure and connectivity, specifically focusing on white matter. Their study examined how "early risky family environments"—characterized by coldness, neglect, and chaos—were associated with weaker white matter integrity in fathers, influencing brain connectivity during the transition to parenthood. Cardenas found that fathers from risky family environments reflect reduced neural connectivity, which in turn predicted less effective parenting (Cardenas et al., 2024). She also referenced their published research on preconception, emphasizing that fathers play a critical yet often overlooked role in shaping offspring outcomes. Saxbe cited Brian Dias's work on pre-conception pathways, reinforcing the idea that fathers contribute to both stress and resilience in significant ways.

DISCUSSION

Reconciling Resilience Research Across Socioeconomic Contexts

Robert Valdez, professor of Family and Community Medicine at the University of New Mexico, asked how to reconcile the finding that socially disadvantaged individuals do not benefit from resilience-building factors as consistently as some datasets suggest. He emphasized the need for integration across studies and highlighted the challenge of defining resilience, questioning whether it should be understood at both societal and individual levels. Rogers emphasized the importance of considering developmental periods when comparing resilience across cohorts, explaining that findings at different ages—such as neonates versus school-aged children or adolescents—may reflect distinct processes in brain development. She cautioned against directly comparing results across studies without accounting for age-related differences in expected neural and behavioral outcomes. She also highlighted a critical factor in her research: Her cohort consists primarily of individuals living below 130 percent of the poverty line, which is a level of disadvantage often underrepresented in resilience studies. Unlike many other datasets, where severely disadvantaged individuals make up a smaller portion of the sample, her cohort's majority population faces extreme socioeconomic hardship, allowing her team to examine resilience in deeply resource-deprived environments. Importantly, Rogers pointed out that when they excluded the most disadvantaged participants, their findings aligned more closely with existing resilience research. However, keeping this highly disadvantaged cohort in the analysis revealed a crucial insight—many conventional resilience factors do not function as expected when fundamental needs such as housing stability, food security, and educational access are not met. She argued that interventions focusing only on individual behavior or parenting strategies are insufficient without addressing the systemic barriers preventing disadvantaged families from benefiting from those efforts. Hyde noted that discrepancies in resilience research could stem from sample-specific factors, particularly the degree of disadvantage. He explained that his lab studies two different cohorts—one facing moderate poverty and another experiencing severe disadvantage—and cautioned that resilience outcomes may depend on where individuals fall on the socioeconomic continuum.

A workshop participant inquired whether research has examined the impacts of overly advantaged neighborhoods on stress resilience. Rogers acknowledged the importance of the question and noted that while some individuals in her studies might fall into the category of being overly advantaged, her research did not specifically analyze this population due to sample limitations. She pointed out that while definitions for social disadvantage and poverty are well established, there is no clear definition for what constitutes being "overly advantaged." Rogers observed that in her research, positive effects of advantage appeared to follow a linear trend, whereas disadvantage showed a threshold effect before leveling off. She concluded that while the question is compelling, she is not aware of any studies directly investigating it.

Peña added that biological heterogeneity plays a role in resilience, emphasizing ongoing research into biomarkers that could help predict individual responses to adversity and improve treatment interventions. Frances Jensen reinforced the importance of biomarkers in resilience research, suggesting that advances in multimodal data may help identify thresholds for resilience and personalize intervention strategies.

Longitudinal Effects of Early Life Stress on Brain Development

Bustamante asked Peña to elaborate on how early life stress shapes neurodevelopment, potentially changing brain circuitry. Peña explained that research over decades has shown early life stress influences development in multiple ways, including altered social, emotional, and cognitive trajectories; changes in amygdala-to-prefrontal cortex connectivity; and delayed developmental milestones in rodents. These varied effects can occur simultaneously rather than being mutually exclusive. She discussed ongoing efforts to study different brain regions, cell types, and gene clusters to better understand these changes. Peña emphasized the importance of a field-wide approach, studying developmental processes longitudinally rather than focusing on single time points in adulthood. She noted that while some outcome measures eventually stabilize, early experiences have lasting effects, and a deeper understanding of brain development during critical periods could inform interventions to realign developmental trajectories.

The Neurological Mechanisms of Context-Specific Resilience

Adding to this perspective, Jensen asked if at different points during the lifespan an individual might develop resilience for one type of stressor but not another, and if this is reflected in the epigenetic changes in rodent models. Meaney cited studies by Gene Brody (e.g., Brody et al., 2013) to highlight how resilience can vary across domains within the same individual or family. He described families in which some members prosper in psychosocial realms (such as stable relationships, academic achievement, and steady employment) while simultaneously displaying vulnerability on biological measures like cardiovascular health and inflammatory responses. Meaney pointed out that these findings challenge a "one-size-fits-all" view of resilience, arguing instead that resilience may be better understood as a pathway-dependent process. He suggested that identifying the specific mediators linking forms of adversity to particular outcomes could provide actionable targets for intervention. Building on this discussion, Hyde noted that while larger brain volume is generally linked to resilience, resilience in children remains highly domain-specific, reinforcing Meaney's argument that resilience follows distinct pathways rather than a universal pattern (Miller-Graff, 2022). Peña acknowledged the complexity of resilience and adversity, explaining that human research is more advanced while rodent studies are still developing. She differentiated between deprivation-related stress (lack of expected experiences) and unpredictable environmental stress and noted that these different types likely influence distinct biological systems depending on the timing of exposure. While rodent models can help disentangle specific effects, she emphasized that in human development, chronic stress makes it difficult to isolate discrete impacts. Peña and Meaney underscored that resilience is not a singular static trait but a dynamic interplay of interdependent processes.

Eric Nestler inquired about brain volume changes in children and adults, asking whether there is a clear pattern of adaptive increases or decreases in brain size across different studies and conditions. Rogers addressed brain volume changes, emphasizing the importance of developmental timing. She noted that early childhood brain growth is expected, but resilience varies across environments—what is adaptive in one setting may be a disadvantage in another. To illustrate this context-dependent resilience, Rogers shared an anecdote from her research on young children in different socioeconomic environments. She explained that her team had difficulty getting two-year-olds to fall asleep in an fMRI scanner for brain imaging. Interestingly, children from more disadvantaged environments—where bedtime routines might have been less rigid—fell asleep more easily. In contrast, children from more structured home environments, who were accustomed to strict bedtime routines and specific comfort items, struggled to fall asleep in the unfamiliar setting. Rogers emphasized how this is just one anecdote that they have observed. Jensen added this might suggest highly structured environments might foster rigidity, potentially making adaptation to unexpected situations more difficult.

Potential Approaches for Resilience-Enhancing Interventions

Deanna Barch, Gregory B. Couch Professor of Psychiatry and vice dean of research at Washington University in St. Louis, asked the panel whether resilience factors, many of which are affected by early adversity, might also serve as optimal targets for intervention. She sought insights into how these mechanisms could guide efforts to promote resilience. Jensen invited Rogers to start the discussion, referencing the THRIVE framework. Rogers noted that their research focuses on identifying the best intervention targets, particularly in caregiver behaviors that influence child resilience. Since neonates cannot actively participate in interventions, the team prioritizes factors within the caregiver's control, including parenting practices, sleep, nutrition, stress reduction, and treatment for mental health conditions. While systemic changes at a societal level would have the greatest impact, Rogers acknowledged that individual families and clinicians will need to work within their immediate environments, as broader societal shifts take time. She emphasized the importance of identifying modifiable mediators—factors individuals can change with the right resources—to effectively promote resilience.

Hyde added to the discussion by highlighting differential susceptibility, referencing research showing that individuals with high amygdala activity tend to thrive with more resources but struggle with fewer. He argued that resilience-building should happen at multiple levels and expressed concern that relying on convenient solutions, such as apps, to address resilience could shift responsibility away from acknowledging and addressing systemic societal issues that contribute to adversity. He stressed that while individual-level interventions are important, scientists must also highlight broader societal influences that shape resilience and ensure that efforts extend beyond what individuals can control. Jensen agreed, emphasizing the need to examine whether structural aspects of society require overhauling or improvement to better support resilience. Rogers pointed to data showing that individuals who lack essential resources do not benefit from conventional resilience-building interventions. She explained that factors like unstable housing, food insecurity, and inadequate education can prevent people from gaining the expected benefits of interventions such as parenting classes. Rogers's evidence supports the argument that resilience cannot be fostered solely at the individual level; systemic issues must also be addressed to create meaningful change.

Nestler wondered how early education programs can increase cognitive function and resilience. In response, Meaney described an early education program in Singapore, an initiative that identifies executive function as a crucial mediator of both risk and resilience, designed to strengthen these skills through structured interventions. Initially, the program faced challenges with implementation—teachers hesitated due to an already packed curriculum. However, once they introduced classroom-based games designed by experts like Clancy Blair, they noticed that students were highly engaged, making the program easier to integrate into daily lessons. Over two to three years, the initiative expanded and is now widely adopted across Singapore's public child care system. The Singapore Ministry of Education's sponsorship played a key role in ensuring the program's success. Ongoing research aims to assess outcomes across multiple domains, including metabolic health, cognitive function, and socioemotional development. Meaney noted that while the games have been shown to work, the next step is to determine which children benefit the most and in what specific ways, refining future interventions accordingly.

On the other hand, Husseini Manji, professor at Oxford University, adjunct professor at Yale University, visiting professor at Duke University, and co-chair of the UK government's Mental Health Goals program, speculated on the role of placebo responses in clinical trials for depression and anxiety. He proposed that some individuals might generate an endogenous resilience process in response to hope and support, potentially influencing treatment outcomes. He brought up the possibility that in preclinical studies environmental enrichment might be an indirect way to enhance endogenous resilience processes. So, perhaps if a treatment worked on top of environmental enrichment, that may increase the likelihood that it would exceed placebo responses in clinical trials.

Andrea Flammia, from Jiayal Media, asked whether there are studies tracking individuals who experienced traumatic childhoods but demonstrated resilience across different life stages. Flammia described experiencing lifelong trauma but building resilience through dance, singing, and music—talents she inherited from her mother. She also highlighted her strong academic performance as further proof of overcoming adversity. She emphasized the need for research examining resilience from biochemical, neural, and environmental perspectives, advocating for greater representation of successful individuals who have overcome adversity. Peña responded by noting that physical activity—particularly dance—has been shown to be a powerful resilience factor in both human and preclinical studies. She highlighted research indicating that dance promotes neurogenesis and plasticity, reinforcing resilience alongside environmental influences such as positive parenting. Flammia followed up by sharing her own academic research on exercise and brain development, expressing excitement over findings that hippocampal volume increases by 12 percent with physical activity. She reiterated the importance of showcasing successful individuals who have navigated adversity, emphasizing that such representation can inspire hope and shift perceptions about long-term outcomes.

Parenting, Emotional Regulation, and Community Responsibility

Another recurrent theme was the interplay between parental mental health and child development. Saxbe discussed the timing of resilience-related brain changes, describing a U-shaped pattern. Prebirth brain-volume decreases appear to be associated with better mental health outcomes, suggesting this reduction may be part of an adaptive process. Postbirth brain-volume increases are also linked to better mental health, indicating recovery and potential resilience following the initial decrease. She emphasized the complexity of modeling these trajectories around sensitive periods. Jon Nelson brought a personal perspective, questioning how long-term exposure to parental mental illness might affect their child's resilience and ability to form authentic interpersonal relationships. Rogers responded by emphasizing the protective role of supportive caregiving. She explained that even when a parent faces chronic challenges, an available emotionally regulated caregiver (which may include the other parent) could buffer adverse effects on the child.

Complementing this view, Meaney highlighted the tendency in literature to attribute poor parenting solely to maternal depression, even though many mothers with depression remain effective caregivers. To support this view, he referenced recent findings by Michelle Kee, which indicate that it is not parental depression itself but the accompanying emotional dysregulation that disrupts child development, as Rogers had mentioned earlier (Kee et al., 2023). Meaney highlighted the importance of targeting emotional regulation in prenatal interventions to better support parenting. Building on Meaney's discussion, Hyde emphasized that parenting behaviors play a more critical role in child outcomes than depression itself. He also addressed broader societal perceptions of mental illness, pointing out that depression is widespread, affecting up to 50 percent of the population, and that mental health struggles are common across families. Hyde stressed that people do not typically choose partners based on whether their parents have mental illnesses, reinforcing the importance of open discussions to normalize these experiences and reduce stigma. He highlighted that such challenges are not abnormal but rather a shared reality for many households. Saxbe drew attention to the idea that resilience is more common than often assumed, explaining that children exposed to parental mental illness or adversity frequently do not experience negative long-term outcomes. She suggested that such experiences could foster empathy and insight within families, contributing to their emotional strength. The dialogue extended to broader societal factors as well: While individual interventions such as parenting classes can be valuable, several panelists pointed to unmet basic needs, such as stable housing, nutrition, and economic security, as critical elements that shape the resilience trajectory.

Emerging Themes in Resilience Research Noted by Workshop Participants

The panelists each offered a brief reflection that encapsulated their views. Terms such as "transformation," "support," "community responsibility," "hope," and "longitudinal intervention" were shared, collectively underscoring the multifaceted, dynamic, and context-dependent nature of resilience across the lifespan. These reflections highlighted that while scientific inquiry continues to unravel the complex biological and environmental influences on development, practical understanding remains rooted in the interplay between individual, familial, and societal resources.

5

The Brain–Body Connection Between Stress Susceptibility and Resilience

Highlights

- Stress affects multiple bodily systems beyond brain function. Early trauma can alter inflammatory cascades, autonomic function, hormone regulation, and microbial communities, thereby predisposing individuals to neuropsychiatric, cardiovascular, and endocrine dysregulation later in life. (Bremner, Gur, Krystal, Montalvo-Ortiz)
- Vagus nerve stimulation could be a promising intervention to improve resilience and physiological regulation. (Bremner)
- Peripheral immune markers, hormonal transport, and blood–brain barrier permeability allow systemic inflammation to impact central processes, raising questions about the complexity of immune regulation and its role in brain health. (Montalvo-Ortiz)
- Stress can alter gut microbial composition, affecting inflammation and neurotransmitter balance—factors linked to psychiatric disorders and the long-term neurodevelopment in infants. Moreover, the microbiome has emerged as a central factor in resilience, with probiotic interventions showing potential to counteract negative effects. (Gur)

NOTE: This list is the rapporteurs' summary of points made by the individual speakers identified, and the statements have not been endorsed or verified by the National Academies of Sciences, Engineering, and Medicine. They are not intended to reflect a consensus among workshop participants.

This chapter shifts the focus to the broader physiological effects of stress, examining its influence on cardiovascular, immune, endocrine, and metabolic functions. Deanna Barch highlighted that stress affects nearly every system in the human body, extending beyond its impact on the brain. She noted that the data presented will illustrate how resilience emerges within these systems and how physiological shifts may shape brain and behavioral outcomes. By exploring these interconnected processes, Barch emphasized the importance of a comprehensive approach to understanding stress susceptibility and resilience.

EPIGENETIC REGULATION AND IMMUNE DYSREGULATION IN STRESS-RELATED OUTCOMES

Janitza Montalvo-Ortiz, assistant professor of psychiatry at Yale University, described the role of epigenetic mechanisms in trauma-related disorders. She began by explaining that epigenetics refers to modifications on DNA—such as DNA methylation, histone modifications, and noncoding RNAs—that alter gene activity without changing the underlying DNA sequence. In DNA methylation, methyl groups attach to specific regions of the DNA (often in gene promoter regions), influencing whether a gene is expressed or is silenced; when present, these modifications usually correlate with decreased gene expression and condensed chromatin (Montalvo-Ortiz et al., 2022). "DNA methylation patterns are established during brain development," she said, and evidence has shown that "childhood trauma can lead to alterations in DNA methylation causing downstream gene expression changes that may influence long-term health and mental health outcomes" (Parade et al., 2021).

Montalvo-Ortiz introduced data from her study, which integrated psychological assessments, epigenetic profiles, and neuroimaging, to illuminate how early life trauma influences long-term mental and physical health. For instance, her team evaluated the methylation of the PCK2 gene, which encodes the mitochondrial phosphoenolpyruvate carboxykinase—a key enzyme driving gluconeogenesis, the process that synthesizes new glucose from noncarbohydrate precursors to sustain stable blood sugar levels when carbohydrate intake is low (Kaufman et al., 2018). PCK2 has been previously linked to an altered methylation pattern that acts as an indirect mediator between childhood trauma and body mass index. Her team focused on OTX2 (orthodenticle homeobox 2), a gene implicated in long-term stress susceptibility, and found that heightened methylation levels predicted higher depression scores among children who had experienced early adversity (Kaufman et al., 2018). Kaufman and colleagues (2018) further linked these epigenetic changes with alterations in neural connectivity—specifically, increased functional connectivity between the ventromedial prefrontal cortex and the anterior cingulate cortex, regions that play a crucial role in emotion regulation.

Beyond peripheral tissue studies, Montalvo-Ortiz referenced some of Michael Meaney's work on postmortem brain samples (Lutz et al., 2017). In donors with a history of childhood abuse, discrete changes in DNA methylation were noted in oligodendrocytes—cells responsible for myelin production—accompanied by downregulation of myelin-related genes and structural alterations in the anterior cingulate cortex, which is important in emotional regulation, cognitive processing, and integrating stress responses. Furthermore, genome-wide approaches investigating DNA methylation in trauma-related disorders have highlighted dysregulation in pathways governing the primary conduit between the brain and peripheral stress responses, the hypothalamic–pituitary–adrenal (HPA) axis, as well as inflammatory processes (Katrinli et al., 2022; Nunez-Rios et al., 2022). Complementary imaging studies using positron emission tomography (PET) have linked lower availability of translocator protein—a microglial marker—with greater post-traumatic stress disorder (PTSD) severity, while peripheral markers of systemic inflammation like C-reactive protein appear to correlate inversely with central immune activity. Collectively, these observations point to a systemic imbalance in immune function, where PTSD appears to drive peripheral inflammation while simultaneously altering neuroimmune responses.

MATERNAL STRESS, THE GUT MICROBIOME, AND INFANT NEURODEVELOPMENT

Tamar Gur, associate professor at The Ohio State University College of Medicine and endowed director of the Sarah Ross Soter Women's Health Research Program, focused on the intricate relationship between maternal stress, gut microbiome composition, and infant neurodevelopment. She explained that during stress the immune system, the HPA axis, and the sympathetic nervous system trigger increases in hormone levels in the gut and intestinal motility, which leads to a disruption in the normal balance of gut microbes—a condition commonly referred to as "dysbiosis" (Gur et al., 2017, 2019).

Under healthy conditions, the gut hosts a complex community of beneficial microorganisms that produce key metabolites. One such metabolite, butyrate—a short chain fatty acid—has significant roles in regulating epigenetic processes. Gur highlighted tryptophan, an essential amino acid obtained solely through diet, which is normally metabolized by specific gut bacteria into beneficial compounds that play key roles in neurodevelopment and immune regulation, such as indole-3-acetic acid and kynurenic acid (Galley et al., 2023, 2024). In experimental models, prenatal stress was shown to reduce the presence of key tryptophan-metabolizing microbes, leading to an altered metabolic profile that could affect the function of microglia, the resident immune cells of the brain known to be critical in synaptic pruning and neurogenesis (see Figure 5-1).

Employing a prenatal mouse model approximately corresponding to the human second trimester with chronic restraint stress, Gur's team demonstrated that even a single episode of maternal stress can set lifelong trajectories in the offspring's microbiome (Gur et al., 2017). Gur assessed variations in the microbial community between experimental groups, revealing distinct shifts in the microbial composition of stressed mouse mothers compared to controls. In parallel, offspring exposed in utero to maternal stress exhibited increased microglial activation—evident by ionized calcium-binding adapter molecule 1 immunolabeling—in the prefrontal cortex. These neuroimmune changes were further paralleled by deficits in social behaviors and, in female animals, heightened anxiety-like behavior.

Integrating clinical findings, Gur referenced a study where pregnant women with elevated anxiety, as measured by the Overall Anxiety Severity and Impairment Scale,[1] transmitted a microbial signature characterized by reduced bifidobacteria dentium to their infants (Galley et al., 2023). Interestingly, experimental supplementation with this microbe in stressed mice led to reductions in interleukin 6 (IL-6) production by microglia and improvements in social behavior (Galley et al., 2024). Such findings underscore the potential for altered microbial profiles to serve as indicators of stress exposure and risk for adverse neurodevelopmental outcomes.

[1] The Overall Anxiety Severity and Impairment Scale is a five-item self-report measure designed to evaluate the severity and functional impact of anxiety across various anxiety disorders. It provides a standardized approach for assessing anxiety-related distress and impairment (Campbell-Sills et al., 2009).

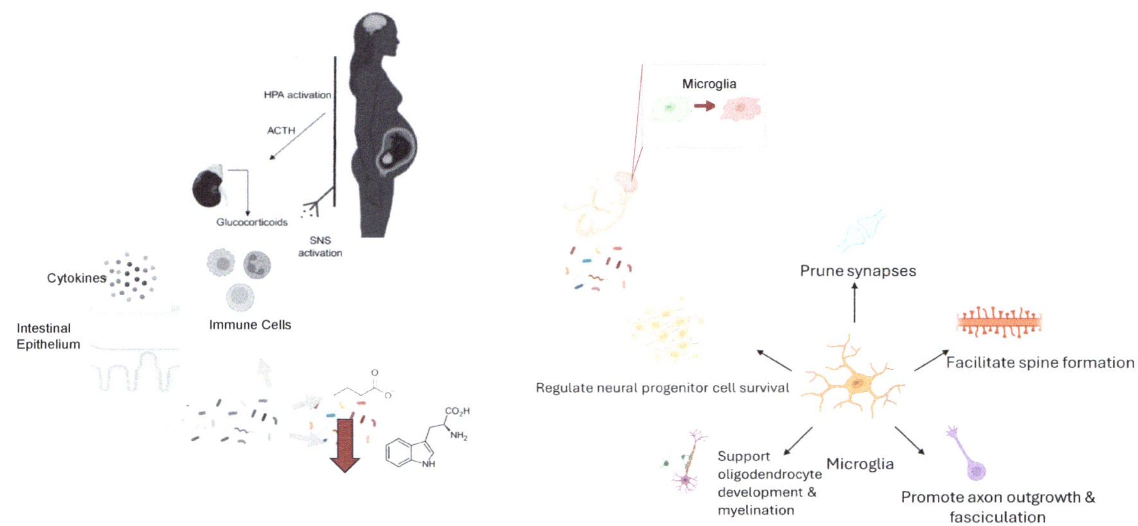

FIGURE 5-1 Illustration of how stress-induced changes activate physiological pathways that can influence the maternal microbiome, which in turn affects the developing fetus.

NOTES: In this process, the interaction between the gut microbiome, immune cells, and tryptophan metabolism is a key factor. More specifically, maternal stress reduces microbes responsible for metabolizing tryptophan, disrupting key neurodevelopmental processes in the fetus. ACTH = adrenocorticotropic hormone; CO2H = carboxyl group; HPA = hypothalamic–pituitary–adrenal axis; NH2 = amino group; O = oxygen; O- = oxygen anion; SNS = sympathetic nervous system.

SOURCE: Presented by Tamar Gur on March 25, 2025.

CARDIOVASCULAR CONSEQUENCES OF STRESS AND BRAIN–HEART COMMUNICATION

Douglas Bremner, professor of psychiatry and radiology at Emory University and director of the Emory Clinical Neuroscience Research Unit, provided insights into how stress and trauma, particularly in PTSD, are interconnected with cardiovascular function. Using data from studies involving Vietnam-era twin pairs, where one twin was exposed to combat and the other was not, Bremner illustrated that stress may precipitate heart problems such as myocardial ischemia even in the absence of extensive atherosclerotic disease, a heart disease marked by fat buildup in the arteries (Moazzami et al., 2020; Vaccarino et al., 2013, 2021, 2022; see Figure 5-2). PET imaging studies revealed reduced heart-related (myocardial) flow reserve, a measure of the heart's ability to increase blood flow under stress conditions, in individuals with elevated PTSD symptoms (Vaccarino et al., 2013).

Bremner emphasized that the altered myocardial blood flow could be linked to changes in autonomic function. Specifically, reduced heart rate variability, particularly in the high-frequency range—a reflection of parasympathetic nervous system activity—is associated with stress-induced myocardial ischemia. Additionally, inflammatory markers, notably IL-6, were observed to show dramatic increases following mental stress tasks (e.g., public speaking challenges and personalized trauma scripts; Vaccarino et al., 2021). These findings point to a scenario in which an overactive sympathetic response, coupled with an inadequate parasympathetic counterbalance, may drive both cardiac dysfunction and heightened inflammatory activity.

The connection between the brain and heart is further exemplified by neuroimaging data. In individuals who exhibited stress-induced ischemia, increased activation in the anterior cingulate and rostromedial prefrontal cortex was detected (Moazzami et al., 2020). These regions are known to process emotions and stress, suggesting that abnormal brain responses could serve as biomarkers for heightened cardiovascular risk. Complementary autonomic measures, such as the pre-ejection period, provided further evidence of sympathetic overdrive during stress. Studies exploring vagus nerve stimulation demonstrated that enhancing parasympathetic activity might attenuate these stress-induced cardiovascular responses, as shown by improvements in myocardial blood flow, stabilized respiratory patterns, and reduced levels of inflammatory cytokines (Bremner et al., 2020). Bremner underscored the profound impact of PTSD and stress on cardiovascular health, highlighting autonomic dysfunction and systemic inflammation as critical mediators of disease progression while presenting vagus nerve stimulation as a promising intervention for both psychological and physiological resilience.

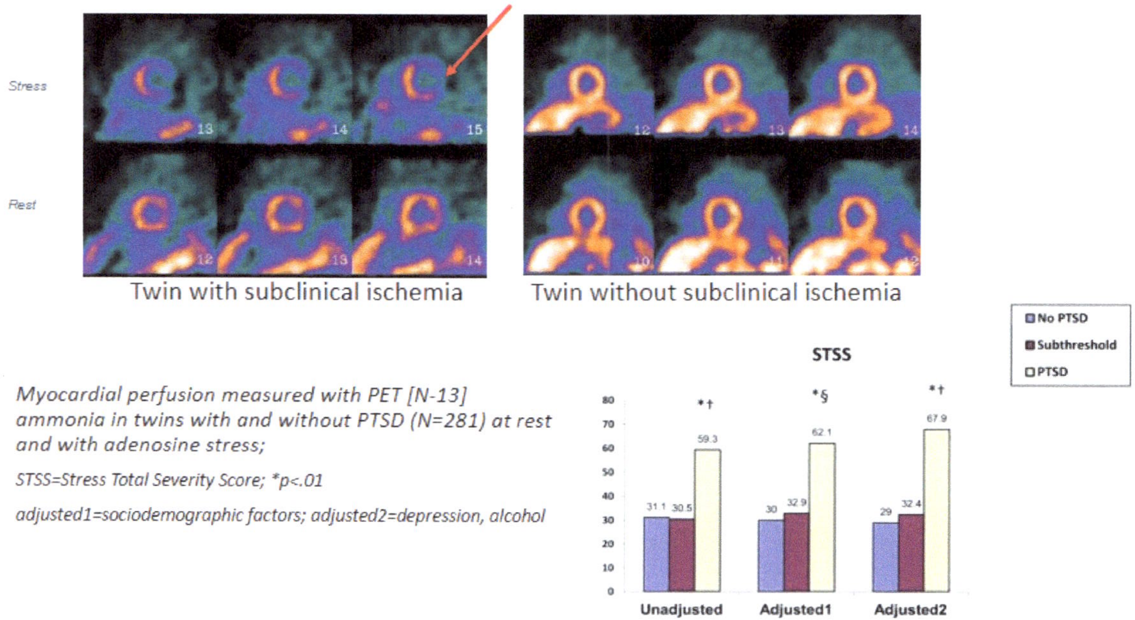

FIGURE 5-2 Negative effects of PTSD on cardiovascular health.
NOTES: Myocardial perfusion was measured using PET in twins with and without PTSD, both at rest and under adenosine-induced stress. PTSD = post-traumatic stress disorder; STSS = Stress Total Severity Score.
SOURCES: Presented by Douglas Bremner on March 25, 2025; adapted from Vaccarino et al., 2013. The scans were created by Viola Vaccarino, and the bar chart is from Vaccarino et al., 2013.

DISCUSSION

Early Adversity and Peripheral Health Outcomes

Nadine Burke Harris shared her curiosity on whether individuals who do not meet criteria for psychopathology but were exposed to early adversity might be linked with adverse peripheral outcomes, such as inflammatory cardiovascular or endocrine dysregulation. Bremner elaborated on this point by noting that although he had previously assumed such outcomes were confined to those with PTSD or other mental health conditions, emerging evidence suggests that early adversity may also manifest in adverse pathophysiology among those without overt clinical disorders. Gur described a pilot study involving 36 women from diverse socioeconomic backgrounds. In these nonpsychiatric participants, her team observed significant relationships between stress, subtle depressive symptoms, and both changes in specific chemokine levels (e.g., CCL2) as well as shifts in the composition of the vaginal and fecal microbiomes (Rajasekera et al., 2024). Bremner later mentioned collaborative work with Rob Anda of the Centers for Disease Control and Prevention that indicated increased cardiovascular risk in broader populations.

John Krystal, chair of psychiatry and the Robert L. McNeil Jr. Professor of Translational Research at Yale University, explained that biological findings can have different implications in psychopathological and nonpsychopathological populations. He referenced studies on Special Forces trainees, noting that while high norepinephrine levels are often associated with pathology in PTSD cases, their meaning depends on accompanying factors, such as neuropeptide Y (NPY) levels (Morgan et al., 2000). Morgan and colleagues (2000) found that resilient trainees exhibited both high norepinephrine and high NPY, suggesting that biological profiles must be interpreted within a broader context when assessing their relationship to psychopathology. Various perspectives pointed to the potential for early life stress to shape peripheral biological and cardiovascular profiles irrespective of psychiatric diagnosis.

Tryptophan Metabolism and Neuropsychiatric Signaling

Kerry Ressler raised a question regarding the role of tryptophan in the broader context of microbiome influences on stress response and if tryptophan could explain some of the individual differences in efficacy of selective serotonin reuptake inhibitors (SSRIs). Gur explained that while tryptophan metabolism is likely one among several mechanisms affected by stress, it may represent a major pathway through which peripheral signals influence the developing brain (Verosky et al., 2025). In her presentation, Gur emphasized not only correlations between stress and altered tryptophan metabolism but also changes in beneficial versus potentially pathogenic microbial populations, especially in historically marginalized populations. Gur presented a nuanced perspective on how tryptophan's interaction with gut health may contribute to individual differences observed in responses to SSRIs. Using pregnancy-related depression as an example, she reaffirmed her stance that treatment is necessary when indicated, as untreated depression itself can negatively affect neurodevelopment. However, Gur raised an important question about whether SSRI treatment might be less effective in individuals with reduced serotonin tryptophan-metabolizing capacity, noting that 95 percent of serotonin is found in the gut rather than the brain. She suggested this area warrants further investigation. Husseini Manji rounded out the discussion by remarking on emerging therapeutic strategies, including targeted immune modulation, and highlighted that while SSRI treatments may alleviate some symptoms of depression, they often do not normalize the diverse biological imbalances observed in stress-related conditions.

The Implications of Blood–Brain Barrier and Gut Permeability for Resilience

Nadine Kabbani, neuroscientist from George Mason University, inquired about the active transport of tryptophan across the blood–brain barrier and whether developmental changes in blood–brain barrier permeability might create periods of heightened vulnerability. While she was less familiar with the blood–brain barrier, she emphasized the placenta's complex role in neurodevelopment and invited further exploration. Montalvo-Ortiz expanded on immune system crosstalk, describing three mechanisms by which peripheral inflammatory signals can enter the brain through the blood–brain barrier: direct active transport, leakage through weak barrier regions, and receptor-mediated transmission. Barch stressed the importance of investigating how stress at different developmental stages affects transport mechanisms and blood–brain barrier function, suggesting further research in offspring. Bremner added insights from single-cell transcriptomic research, noting that vascular endothelial cells show changes in PTSD, including shifts in cell adhesion molecules, which could indicate altered blood–brain barrier permeability in adults.

Complementary to this dialogue, Brian Dias introduced the idea of extracellular vesicles as an alternative mechanism of communication across biological barriers—thus broadening the discussion to consider nontraditional carriers of biological signals beyond immune function and hormone signaling. Montalvo-Ortiz acknowledged the complexity of the question and speculated on how hormones might cross the blood–brain barrier, highlighting the role of HPA-axis activation in peripheral inflammatory signaling. Regarding extracellular vesicles, tiny carriers of molecular signals, Gur highlighted research led by Banu Gumusoglu at the University of Iowa, which examines their role in preterm birth. She noted that severe depression during pregnancy has been linked to preterm birth, a relationship that may or may not be mitigated by antidepressant treatment (Gumusoglu, 2024). Gur suggested that extracellular vesicles could play a key role in transmitting stress-related biological information between mother and offspring. She reflected on previous assumptions in the maternal immune activation field, where it was believed that inflammation in the mother directly led to inflammation in the offspring. However, her research indicates that this is not necessarily the case for stress-related signaling. Instead, she proposed that extracellular vesicles might serve as crucial mechanisms in this process, potentially shaping fetal development and stress susceptibility. Barch underscored the importance of examining these permeability mechanisms developmentally, noting the need for more research on how stress at different time points impacts transport mechanisms and regulatory systems.

Laura Bustamante shared insights from her personal experience with fructose malabsorption and its impact on her mental health and mood, which brought attention to the promise of dietary and probiotic interventions as vehicles for mitigating stress-induced microbiome alterations. Gur pointed out the lack of discussion on gut permeability, expanding the discussion beyond the blood–brain barrier to include gut permeability and placental function. She noted that gut permeability, often referred to in discussions of "leaky gut," has implications for both individual health and intergenerational effects. Disorders such as irritable bowel syndrome and inflammatory bowel disease frequently co-occur with psychiatric conditions, raising questions about the interplay between gut permeability, stress, and mental health. Gur pointed out that stress-induced permeability changes may not only affect the individual but could also have consequences for the next generation, potentially influencing neurodevelopmental outcomes. She also referenced research on extracellular vesicles in relation to preterm birth, linking them to maternal stress signaling and the broader question of how biological information is transmitted from mother to offspring.

The Intersection of Inflammation and Mental Health

Andrew Fuligni, professor of psychology and psychiatry at the University of California, Los Angeles, asked about the challenges in assessing neuroimmune functioning across development. He wondered how best to conceptualize healthy versus unhealthy immune states in infants, children, and adolescents when most available models are derived from adult populations. Gur and Montalvo-Ortiz pointed out that measures taken from adult populations may not directly translate to younger individuals. Montalvo-Ortiz agreed that there is no clear consensus on immune function, even in adults, especially concerning PTSD and developmental psychopathology. She discussed the variability in immune signaling across different biological systems, highlighting inconsistencies in pro-inflammatory markers and neuroimmune suppression in PTSD. She also highlighted the complexity of IL-6, which has both pro-inflammatory and anti-inflammatory effects, depending on its role in the brain and periphery. As research expands beyond peripheral markers to brain-specific immune function, she emphasized the need for further exploration of these relationships across development. Gur acknowledged the complexity of Fuligni's question and expanded on the topic by discussing pregnancy as another critical period of immune changes. She emphasized the lack of a clear definition of normal immune function across the lifespan, particularly regarding the microbiome and immune markers. Gur noted that without a full understanding of what constitutes a healthy microbiome, defining immune dysfunction remains challenging.

Herman Taylor observed that the mortality curves for patients with PTSD and stress-induced myocardial ischemia were reminiscent of those seen in studies of post-myocardial-infarction depression. In his remarks, Taylor queried whether interventions in the psychiatric domain might have measurable effects on cardiovascular outcomes and whether these outcomes might ultimately depend on addressing underlying inflammatory processes. Bremner recalled past trials—such as the Enhancing Recovery in Coronary Heart Disease (ENRICHD) study (Writing Committee for the ENRICHD Investigators, 2003)—and acknowledged that interventions for depression have yielded only modest benefits in terms of cardiovascular endpoints. Complementing these clinical insights, Krystal remarked that the relationship between systemic inflammation and mental health is intricate; the presence of depression may sometimes serve as a biomarker of a broader inflammatory state rather than acting as an isolated causal factor. Huda Akil added to the conversation by emphasizing that individual variability in biological responses (including differences in insulin resistance and microbiome composition) could help explain why some individuals are more vulnerable than others to the cascading effects of stress. As a unifying theme, Gur invoked a Greek phrase that links mental and physical well-being, "a sound mind and a sound body," suggesting that a harmonious balance between the two is critical even if such a balance is challenging to achieve in practice.

Montalvo-Ortiz highlighted the rapid advancement of bioinformatics tools in helping researchers analyze and interpret complex datasets. She discussed efforts to disentangle cause from consequence in the role of inflammatory signaling in PTSD, citing studies that use polygenic risk scores of inflammatory markers from large datasets like the UK Biobank. She also noted that methods such as Mendelian randomization[2] are being employed to explore mediation mechanisms and causality. As data and analytical tools continue to evolve, Montalvo-Ortiz emphasized their potential to enhance understanding of the biological factors underlying stress susceptibility.

Workshop participants discussed the profound interconnectedness of stress with physiological systems, demonstrating its impact on neuroimmune function, cardiovascular health, metabolism, and microbiome regulation. As research advances, integrating perspectives from psychiatry, immunology, and neuroscience may help develop targeted interventions that promote resilience across both mental and physical health.

[2] Mendelian randomization is a research method that uses genetic differences people inherit from their parents to help scientists determine whether certain environmental factors directly cause health effects rather than just being associated with them. This approach helps researchers make stronger conclusions about cause and effect in health studies (Smith and Ebrahim, 2003).

6

Public Health and Clinical Strategies to Enhance Resilience

Highlights

- Although often overlooked in traditional stress research, positive experiences and human adaptability play an important role in resilience-building, and exploring mechanisms that both reduce the impact of negative experiences and enhance responsiveness to positive ones might offer greater insight into human functioning and adaptability. (Fuligni)
- Adverse childhood experiences (ACEs) constitute a public health crisis with immense societal costs. Expanding treatment access to individuals at high risk of having a toxic stress physiology with an ACE score of four or more regardless of mental health diagnosis has demonstrated improved access to care, quality of care, and outcomes along with potentially significant cost saving compared to traditional reactive care models. (Burke Harris)
- Longitudinal studies reveal that chronic exposure to racial discrimination, economic instability, and neighborhood disadvantage accelerates aging and increases disease susceptibility, disproportionately affecting Black communities and contributing to rising suicide rates among Black youth. Equipping parents with cultural strategies that foster racial pride not only reduces depressive symptoms in youth but also recalibrates neural

responses that can collectively strengthen lifelong resilience. (McBride Murry)
- Despite the complexity of symptoms observed in children who have experienced abuse and neglect, a thorough holistic assessment can lead to clear, focused, and personalized treatment pathways that are effective and responsive to each child's unique circumstances. (Minnis)
- Families can play a key role in protecting their children from the negative consequences of adversity, but masking underlying physiological stress can lead to onset of early aging. As such, there is a need for broader structural-level interventions beyond family, individual, and community support to alleviate the hidden mental, behavioral, and physical health burdens of discrimination and poverty. (Burke Harris, McBride Murry)
- While adverse experiences pose risks, many individuals have the capacity to adapt when provided with proper support. Reframing trauma as a challenge rather than an inevitable determinant of negative outcomes fosters empowerment and allows affected individuals to develop resilience through structured interventions and relational networks. (Burke Harris, Minnis)

NOTE: This list is the rapporteurs' summary of points made by the individual speakers identified, and the statements have not been endorsed or verified by the National Academies of Sciences, Engineering, and Medicine. They are not intended to reflect a consensus among workshop participants.

Andrew Fuligni referenced Huda Akil's discussion on the rise of mental distress among young people, suggesting that increasing stress levels may be worsened by a diminished emphasis on positive experiences, fewer opportunities for meaningful engagement, or an underutilization of neural systems designed to respond to such experiences. He proposed that as negativity escalates, access to enriching and supportive experiences may decline, further compounding the issue. Fuligni encouraged deeper exploration into mechanisms that not only mitigate the effects of negative experiences but also actively enhance responsiveness to positive ones. He also underscored the importance of resilience-building systems linked to positive experiences and human adaptability—elements often overlooked in traditional discussions of stress. This chapter, therefore, centers on the application of biological and clinical insights into stress and resilience to strengthen public health strategies in intervention, prevention, and the detection of stress-related effects.

EVIDENCE-BASED MECHANISMS FOR EARLY INTERVENTION AND PUBLIC AWARENESS

Nadine Burke Harris discussed the profound public health implications of ACEs and toxic stress, framing these issues as a pressing public health crisis. She highlighted that two-thirds of the population have at least one ACE, but these experiences are disproportionately distributed among marginalized communities (Merrick et al., 2019). The term ACE originates from a landmark study conducted by the Centers for Disease Control and Prevention (CDC) and Kaiser Permanente over two decades ago (Felitti et al., 1998). The study identified 10 key categories of stressful or traumatic childhood events (see Figure 6-1). ACEs are preventable, potentially traumatic experiences that occur before the age of 18 and are linked to a wide range of negative health outcomes. Understanding these categories helps inform prevention and intervention strategies aimed at reducing their long-term impact. Burke Harris's discussion elaborated on the dose-response relationships observed between ACE exposure and a range of adverse outcomes, with the greatest health risk associated with four or more ACEs (Putnam et al., 2013). These include associations with mental health conditions, substance use, homelessness, childhood adversity, and even links with the 10 leading causes of death.[1]

The CDC recently published a study estimating the annual economic burden of ACEs in the United States at approximately $14.1 trillion in direct health care costs and lost productivity (Peterson et al., 2023). Recognizing the scale of this impact, discussions have increasingly centered on the need to understand the biology of adversity to inform targeted public health strategies. Burke Harris reflected on earlier workshop discussions about how the biological effects of early life stress extend across multiple systems, such as the epigenetic, inflammatory, and endocrine pathways. Key disruptions include alterations in the hypothalamic–pituitary–adrenal axis, alongside impacts on critical brain regions such as the amygdala, prefrontal cortex, hippocampus, and the ventral tegmental area involved in reward processing. Burke Harris also noted that there is an increasing amount of evidence that stress can be treated (Bick et al., 2015; Chino and Debruyn, 2006; Miller et al., 2014).

[1] According to the CDC's National Center for Health Statistics, the leading causes of death in the United States in 2022 included heart disease, cancer, accidents (unintentional injuries), COVID-19, stroke (cerebrovascular diseases), chronic lower respiratory diseases, Alzheimer's disease, diabetes, nephritis (including nephrotic syndrome and nephrosis), and chronic liver disease and cirrhosis (Kochanek et al., 2022).

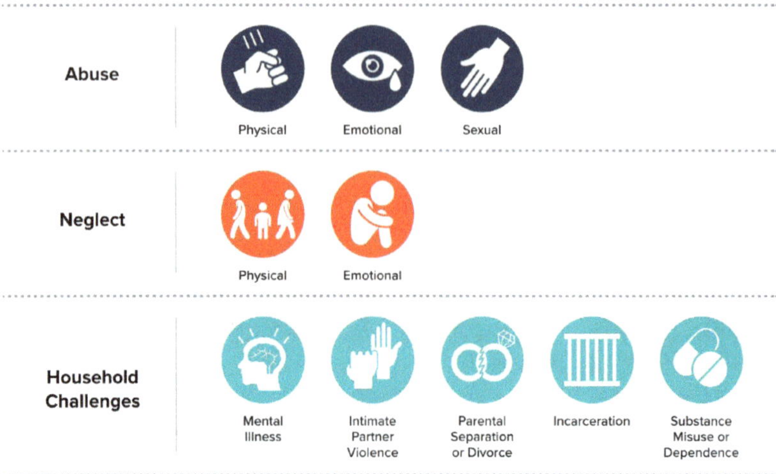

FIGURE 6-1 Categories of adverse childhood experiences (ACEs).
NOTE: ACEs, identified in a CDC–Kaiser Permanente study, refer to 10 types of traumatic childhood events in three categories: Abuse (physical, emotional, or sexual); neglect (physical or emotional); and household dysfunction (parental incarceration, mental illness, substance dependence, divorce, or intimate partner violence).
SOURCES: Presented by Nadine Burke Harris on March 25, 2025; adapted from the Office of the California Surgeon General, 2025.

Burke Harris shared her efforts in helping to launch California's Initiative to Advance Precision Medicine, a groundbreaking first-in-the-nation effort in toxic stress research, by focusing on the early detection of adversity's effects on brain, immune, hormonal, and thymic development during critical periods to improve outcomes. Primary care providers were trained to screen universally for ACEs not merely to document history but to assess risk for a dysregulated physiologic stress response. Burke Harris noted, "For those who are at high risk of having a toxic stress response, we implement evidence-based interventions to regulate the stress physiology."

One example of an evidence-based intervention is a University of California, Los Angeles, pilot study that examined the effectiveness of virtual mindfulness interventions in children screened for ACEs. Participants demonstrated measurable reductions in symptoms, as indicated by improvements in their Patient Health Questionnaire-9 scores—a widely used depression screening tool. This study underscored the value of accessible nonclinical interventions that directly target physiological stress responses before they progress into more severe mental health conditions.

Additionally, Burke Harris discussed California's policy shift, which expanded eligibility criteria for wraparound services based on the evidence and the science of toxic stress. Previously, children required a formal diagnosis of a mental health disorder to receive support. However, under new guidelines, children with an ACE score of four or more could qualify based on their risk level alone. This approach enabled earlier detection through interventions such as the California Advancing and Innovating Medi-Cal (CalAIM) program[2] during critical developmental periods, potentially preventing long-term health consequences associated with toxic stress. The impact of this policy change was profound, dramatically increasing the number of children eligible for enhanced care management, substance use treatment, and mental health support. Burke Harris stressed that this model, currently implemented in California, could serve as a framework for other states or countries seeking to mitigate the intergenerational cycle of ACEs and stress-related health outcomes.

Building on these systemic efforts to address toxic stress, First 5 California[3] launched a $120 million public education campaign that led to a 2.5-fold increase in community awareness of both toxic stress and ACEs, with 89 percent of respondents believing in the potential for children to heal from trauma and 88 percent confident in breaking the cycle of toxic stress. In parallel, a youth-designed campaign emerged, where messages crafted by young people for their peers resonated more effectively, highlighting the benefits of tailored, age-specific communication in supporting efforts to disrupt this cycle.

CLINICAL INTERVENTIONS AND PUBLIC HEALTH STRATEGIES PROMOTING RESILIENCE

Velma McBride Murry, university distinguished professor in the Department of Health Policy at the Vanderbilt School of Medicine and Department of Human and Organizational Development at Vanderbilt University, shared that the alarming 233 percent increase in suicide rates among Black youth over the last decade is a significant issue that highlights the need for greater public awareness and engagement from policymakers, researchers, and community leaders to identify and eliminate the root cause of lost lives among Black youth (Sheftall, 2023). This trend points to the need for thoughtful discussion and

[2] CalAIM is an initiative to improve care and outcomes for millions of Medi-Cal enrollees. It is led by the California Department of Health Care Services. CalAIM builds on prior initiatives, like the Whole Person Care pilots, Health Homes program, Drug Medi-Cal Organized Delivery System, and the Coordinated Care Initiative. See https://calaim.dhcs.ca.gov/ (accessed July 18, 2025).

[3] First 5 California is an initiative that aims to establish a comprehensive, integrated, and coordinated system to benefit California's youngest children and their families, with a core mandate to enhance early childhood health, education, and family resilience (California First 5, 2025).

a deeper examination of contributing factors beyond the individual or family circumstances. McBride Murry highlighted that, although discussions of youth mental health disparities often take a broad approach, Black youth specifically experience an exceptionally high and disproportionate increase in suicide rates at younger ages (Sheftall, 2023). This troubling pattern, she underscored, requires interventions that address not only individual behaviors but also the broader structural and system level that has historically perpetuated a wide array of disparities.

McBride Murry introduced the concept of syndemic conditions, explaining that multiple interrelated stressors—including racial discrimination, neighborhood disadvantage, and economic instability—work together to compound health disparities, leading to early mortality and chronic disease (Lei et al., 2022). She pointed to evidence showing that 44 percent of ACEs are preventable, suggesting that reducing exposure to these conditions could significantly impact long-term health trajectories. Rather than viewing adversity in isolation, she framed syndemic conditions as systemic, reinforcing cycles of harm over generations.

Recognizing the continued need for systemic change, McBride Murry highlighted family-level interventions as part of the broader approach to mitigate adversities. McBride Murry pointed to the benefit of a racial-equity-affirming parenting program, a protective process targeted in the Pathways for African American Success (PAAS), designed to enhance parenting skills to foster resilience in their children. Racial-equity-affirming parenting is a socialization process by which parents equip their children with strategies to navigate adversity, particularly in the context of environments where they are at greater risk for experiencing racial stress and discrimination. PAAS-induced racial-equity-affirming parenting demonstrated significant reductions in depressive symptoms among participating youth, even in the presence of racial discrimination.

This finding highlighted the protective role of culturally attuned parenting practices in buffering children from racialized adversities. McBride Murry also shared findings from a recent study, testing the extent to which PAAS enhanced brain functionality. This is the first study to merge prevention and neuroscience in a test of the effectiveness of a family-strength-based program to increase cognitive, emotional, and self-regulation behaviors among youth by enhancing both caregiver and youth protective processes. Findings revealed that youth assigned to the PAAS program demonstrated greater increases on neuronal coupling of the ventral striatum and ventrolateral prefrontal cortex, brain regions associated with improved risk resistance coping skills, compared to youth assigned to waitlist control (Gillespie et al., 2020). Furthermore, results shed light on the importance of enhancing regions of the brain that influence optimal decision making, self-regulation, and emotional coping to

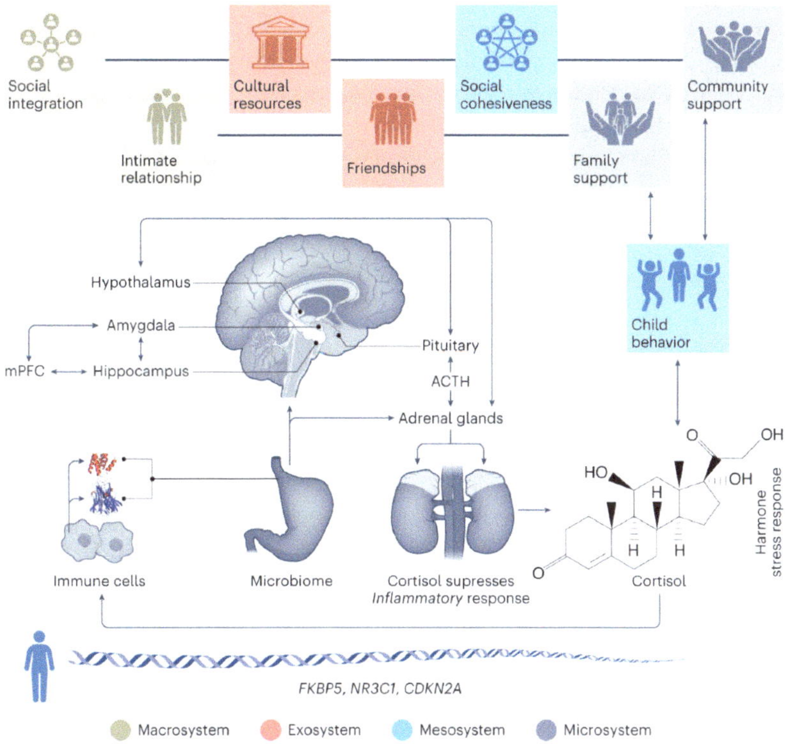

FIGURE 6-2 The bio-exposome represents the dynamic links across molecular, physiological, clinical, and societal levels.
NOTE: ACTH = adrenocorticotropic hormone; mPFC = medial prefrontal cortex; FKBP5 = FK506 binding protein 5; NR3C1 = nuclear receptor subfamily 3 group C member 1; CDKN2A = cyclin dependent kinase inhibitor 2A; O = oxygen; H = hydrogen; OH = hydroxyl group.
SOURCES: Presented by Helen Minnis on March 25, 2025; adapted from Minnis et al., 2024.

prepare youth to navigate adversities, particularly challenges that elevate risk vulnerabilities.

In her final comments, McBride Murry added that merging findings from the brain functioning testing of PAAS to two of her other studies on the promotion of racial-equity-informed parenting and racial pride, noting that these studies collectively may offer insights on the importance of greater insight on how the protective nature of brain development in the midst of adversity. Being equipped with coping strategies through culturally attuned parental socialization may provide an environment to enhance awareness, and improve neural responses when processing environmental cues. These cues are processed cognitively and emotionally, giving signals of how to respond in that manner that reduces hypervigilance and threat. This shift in attentional processing may contribute to reduced anxiety and stress-related disorders later in life. Altogether, McBride Murry's findings underscored the need for systemic approaches integrating neuroscience and public health efforts to disrupt cycles of adversity and promote long-term well-being.

OPTIMISM IN TREATMENT AMONG COMPLEXITIES IN CHILDHOOD ABUSE

Helen Minnis, a professor of child and adolescent psychiatry at the University of Glasgow, explored the need for better assessments of the complex interplay between childhood abuse and neglect and later mental health outcomes. Minnis began by noting that although abuse and neglect increase the risk of psychiatric issues, the global picture is not straightforward (Vila-Badia et al., 2021). For instance, epidemiological maps suggest that regions like sub-Saharan Africa, where exposure to abuse is reportedly high, do not necessarily show parallel rates of conditions such as schizophrenia, as seen in North America (Fernandes et al., 2021; Solmi et al., 2023). This contrast raises intriguing questions about the direct links between early adversity and later psychiatric disorders.

Delving into the science of early trauma, Minnis discussed research that emphasizes children's biological capacity to adapt to adverse conditions. She referenced the Adaptive Calibration Model of Stress Responsivity—a framework that accounts for individual differences in stress responsivity as shaped by early environments and evolving across the lifespan—highlighting the idea that "children have evolved…to respond in biologically adaptive ways to harsh and unsupportive family environments, not just loving and supportive ones" (Del Giudice et al., 2011). These physiological adaptations can help children function in challenging contexts and may partly explain why some children exposed to severe abuse or neglect do not inevitably develop mental health problems. However, the model also recognizes that such adaptations occur within a broader context of risk, and adverse outcomes can still emerge, especially when environmental demands exceed the limits of these evolved coping mechanisms.

Expanding on this theme, Minnis introduced the concept of the "bio-exposome" (see Figure 6-2). This framework captures the dynamic interactions among genetic predispositions, stress regulation, immune responses, the microbiome, neural development, and the broader social environment (Minnis et al., 2024). Using the example of a child reacting to traumatic experiences with elevated cortisol levels and observable externalizing behaviors, she illustrated how these early indicators could potentially steer life trajectories. In environments where supportive interventions or naturally nurturing relationships emerge, the outlook may shift toward more positive social and developmental outcomes.

Another key point discussed was the complexity seen in neurodevelopmental profiles among children who have experienced abuse and neglect. Drawing on her clinical observations and a large twin study from Sweden, Minnis noted that children with early maltreatment were six times more likely to exhibit multiple neurodevelopmental conditions such as attention-deficit/hyperactivity disorder, autism, tic disorders, and learning disabilities (Minnis, 2013). Although Minnis initially thought that maltreatment was causing the heightened comorbidity among neurodevelopmental conditions, her findings pointed to additional genetic factors that might predispose the children to additional neurodevelopmental conditions. While the study could not explain what those genetic factors are, it raised the possibility that these factors may reflect neurodevelopmental conditions that run in families. If a child presents with such a condition, it is conceivable that the child's parents might also experience heritable challenges in learning, impulse control, language, or social understanding. This perspective offers a measure of optimism, as the well-established support for neurodevelopmental conditions in both children and adults could hold promise in mitigating the impact of ACEs.

Minnis emphasized the importance of assessing abused and neglected children with respect for their journey, as earlier mentioned by Akil. She referenced a collaborative effort led by Rachel Hiller, in which international clinical academics examined how to approach such assessments. Their key finding was that despite the complexity of abused or neglected children's experiences and needs, the underlying mental health symptoms requiring treatment are often straightforward (Hiller et al., 2023). Minnis noted that a holistic assessment can help identify these core issues, allowing for a clear and focused treatment approach.

Minnis underscored the urgent need to provide children who have experienced neglect or abuse with comprehensive assessments that form the foundation for high-quality, individualized care. Moreover, she reinforced the shared perspective among workshop presenters that resilience is not a static trait but a journey. She emphasized that both children and adults burdened by ACEs require steadfast compassionate support to empower them toward genuine thriving.

DISCUSSION

Economic Impacts in Early Intervention Strategies

Catherine Jensen Peña asked a question centered on the financial viability of early intervention programs that seek to prevent ACEs before they manifest as full-fledged clinical conditions. Burke Harris explained that since launching the initiative in 2020, her team has been examining data spread across various systems. The previous estimated lifetime impact of ACEs on direct health care cost was $124 billion, and the new estimate provided by the CDC rose to $14.1 trillion annually. Burke Harris pointed out that a significant portion of these expenses derives from costly conditions such as cardiovascular diseases and that even after accounting for traditional risk behaviors, biological factors—specifically, a dysregulated stress response combined with neuroendocrine and immune disruptions—continue to elevate risk for chronic conditions. This is in drastic contrast to the cost analysis of California's coordinated public health approach, which estimated an annual cost of roughly $112.5 billion on California's health care system. This contrast suggests that addressing only symptomatic diseases might result in interventions that are not only costly but only partially effective, compared to the cost-effective preventive approach.

Brian Dias inquired about the eligibility criteria for public health programs such as Medi-Cal, specifically whether children with four or more ACEs qualify independently of traditional eligibility requirements. Burke Harris explained that children at high risk for toxic stress are eligible for CalAIM under a clinical algorithm that assesses ACE scores, ACE-related health conditions, and family protective factors. She noted that a child with four or more ACEs who does not have a mental health diagnosis may not necessarily require care from a licensed mental health professional. To address the broader need for stress regulation, Burke Harris highlighted California's efforts to train and expand the capacity of community-based organizations in evidence-based interventions—such as sleep, exercise, nutrition, mindfulness, mental health support, and healthy relationships. These initiatives are designed to be culturally and linguistically appropriate, helping to reduce the burden on the state's mental health providers while increasing access to community-based care.

The "Rubber Suit" Metaphor: Cultural Resilience in Context

Simone Gentilhomme, a master's student in social work at Howard University, introduced a metaphorical inquiry by asking about the notion of the "rubber suit" (Murry et al., 2023). McBride Murry came up with the concept of the "rubber suit" while looking at protective gear during the COVID-19 pandemic (see Figure 6-3). It represents the socially inculcated coping mechanisms that Black families use to face toxic social and environmental challenges. In her depiction, optimism functions as the essential goggles—sharpening vision with hope and a forward-looking perspective—while the kinship system becomes a sturdy backpack, laden with the indispensable support of extended family and community. Racial pride acts as an antibacterial spray

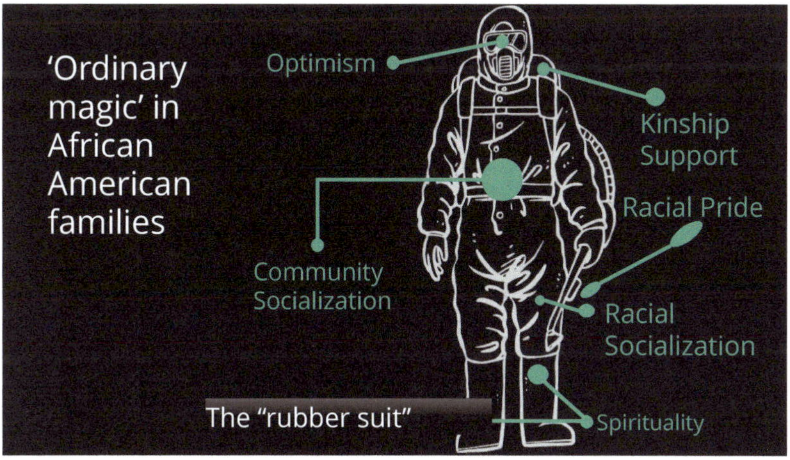

FIGURE 6-3 Rubber suit metaphor illustrating the protective gear Black family members rely on to navigate the challenges of society.
SOURCES: Presented by Velma McBride Murry on March 25, 2025; adapted from Murry et al., 2023.

bottle, offsetting negative societal messages, and community socialization ties everything together like a reliable belt that holds the system in place. Finally, spirituality serves as the grounding boots, enabling individuals to advance steadily despite persistent systemic challenges. Together, these elements form a comprehensive, ever-adaptable defense—embodying both the resilience and the inevitable burdens of safeguarding oneself within systems marked by adversity. In response to Gentilhomme on her inquiry using McBride Murry's metaphor of a "too-tight rubber suit" to describe clients overwhelmed by their own coping systems, Burke Harris emphasized that risk factors for developing the toxic stress response extend well beyond childhood maltreatment to include systemic factors like discrimination and poverty.

Dias questioned how the rubber suit metaphor accounts for "skin-deep resilience," where outward displays of strength may mask underlying biological weathering, including inflammation. Minnis responded by underscoring the importance of family and community in fostering resilience, particularly in societies that have become increasingly nuclear. She reflected on the vital role of extended family networks—such as support from aunties, grandparents, and cousins as seen in Caribbean cultures—in buffering stress and promoting well-being. Minnis argued that in nuclear societies, individuals may experience a different kind of biological weathering, as they often face adversity alone rather than within a strong communal support system. She stressed that marginalized communities, which traditionally rely on extended family structures, possess strengths that should be recognized and integrated into broader societal frameworks. Minnis advocated for surrounding children and young people with these extended support systems to help recalibrate their physiological responses to stress and enhance resilience.

McBride Murry expanded the conversation by considering resilience in the context of intergenerational survival and genetic inheritance. She pointed to historical examples, such as the survival of individuals during the transatlantic slave trade, suggesting that genetic and environmental factors have been transmitted across generations, contributing to intergenerational resilience. McBride Murry questioned how resilience traits might be "transported" from ancestors to the present, shaping how individuals navigate adversity today. She summarized findings from a longitudinal study of more than 800 families participating in the Family and Community Health Study, which has tracked both risk and protective processes in African American families since the early 1990s. Findings from McBride Murry and her colleagues have shown that despite generational poverty, families consistently exhibit protective mechanisms as pathways for their children to thrive. McBride Murry also raised concerns about the burdens placed on parents to "be resilient" so that their children will be healthy, arguing that greater attention should be given to supporting caregivers so that *they* are healthy and able to effectively nurture resilient children. Husseini Manji added to the conversation by highlighting the importance of caregiver support and the positive role of extended family structures in mental health outcomes, particularly in conditions like schizophrenia.

Understanding Trauma in a Complex Societal Context

Akil questioned whether the rising prevalence of mental health issues might be understood through a lens like the "hygiene hypothesis," suggesting that just as exposure to microbes is integral to immune system functioning, a balanced engagement with life's challenges might be necessary for building robust resilience. She wondered whether reduced exposure to adversity in some populations might contribute to rising depression rates. Minnis found the question intriguing but acknowledged the complexity of resilience. She pointed to historical contexts where shared experiences of hardship fostered social support, contrasting this with modern societies in which trauma can lead to increased fragility due to social isolation. While she recognized ongoing inequalities, she also suggested that some communities may have become overly insulated from adversity. Burke Harris challenged the idea that reduced exposure to adversity is a cause of rising depression rates. Instead, she framed trauma as an unavoidable part of life, much like microbial exposure. She emphasized that ACEs significantly increase the risk of numerous health conditions and argued that interventions often fail when they only address symptoms rather than the underlying dysregulated stress response. Christopher Weber, director of Global Science Initiatives at the Alzheimer's Association, expanded on the discussion by drawing connections between structural inequities—such as interpersonal racism and neighborhood disadvantages—and later-life cognitive challenges.

Laura Bustamante praised the ACEs program, which provides children exposed to toxic stress with mental health support without conferring psychiatric diagnosis. She shared her personal experiences, reflecting on how despite being "a really resilient, really positive kid," she believes she would have benefited from such a program. Burke Harris warned against overlooking the physiological consequences of trauma and advocated for a broader systemic approach to treatment. She underscored that while interventions at the individual level are valuable, transformative change also requires bolstering community relationships and cultivating societal infrastructure that nurtures healing.

Digital Mental Health Solutions

A workshop participant wondered about digital technology's potential to scale supportive interventions, such as using AI and mental health chatbots. McBride Murry revisited her earlier research and described an electronic health version of a family-based preventive intervention program that was deployed across multiple digital platforms. She suggested that these methods may allow communities even in rural areas to access evidence-based approaches for regulating stress responses. In discussing digital literacy and the use of AI-driven mental health chatbots, McBride Murry noted that care must be taken to ensure these digital tools incorporate diverse cultural and linguistic perspectives. The conversation highlighted a vision of "virtual villages" where digital platforms serve as extensions of community-based care, helping to bridge gaps in access and support.

Bridging Research and Practice for Broader Societal Change

Throughout this chapter, workshop speakers highlighted the importance of identifying adverse experiences early to facilitate intervention and treatment. Negative factors such as racial discrimination, economic instability, and neighborhood disadvantage can cause severe physiological stress and aging. But strong, warm support systems have been repeatedly demonstrated to alleviate some of the biological burden of adverse experiences. Early interventions have also been demonstrated to not only improve health outcomes but also decrease the economic burden, which could be the target of public health and advocacy initiatives.

7

Advancing Resilience Research: Key Insights and Potential Next Steps

Highlights

- Broader influences, including workplace stress and rapid societal changes, are unexplored key factors that may interact with biological and behavioral elements of resilience, underscoring the importance of incorporating these external stressors into research and intervention strategies. (Jensen, Nestler)
- Biomarkers, behavioral indicators, and computational modeling provide critical insights into resilience-related brain circuits, helping rapidly test new hypotheses and define predictive markers for resilience. (Jensen, Vicentic)
- Redefining resilience as a dynamic biological trait with far-reaching intergenerational effects forces the field to rethink how resilience is measured. (Akil, Krystal, Nelson)
- Personal narratives and metaphors illustrated that stress recovery is an ongoing process and highlighted concerns that disruptions in underlying mechanisms could lead to "diseases of resilience," where even treatments might inadvertently affect recovery trajectories. (Krystal, Nelson)

- Interventions such as pretreatment with N-methyl-D-aspartate (NMDA) antagonists (e.g., ketamine) and the use of lithium not only provide acute symptom relief but also appear to enhance synaptic plasticity and bolster long-term resilience through molecular pathways. (Manji)

NOTE: This list is the rapporteurs' summary of points made by the individual speakers identified, and the statements have not been endorsed or verified by the National Academies of Sciences, Engineering, and Medicine. They are not intended to reflect a consensus among workshop participants.

Eric Nestler highlighted the workshop's exploration of key topics, including the biological foundations of stress responses with an emphasis on resilience, critical developmental periods, and the bidirectional interaction between peripheral organs and the brain in regulating stress susceptibility. He also acknowledged discussions on the broader societal and policy implications of this research. This chapter examines gaps in knowledge and considers where resources may be allocated to enhance resilience and mitigate the negative effects of stress on society.

LEVERAGING BIOLOGICAL MECHANISMS FOR EARLY DETECTION AND INTERVENTION

Aleksandra Vicentic outlined how studies on stress-mediated changes in neuroplasticity (the brain's ability to reorganize itself) have illuminated sensitive periods of risk and resilience during development. She described how employing quantitative behavioral tasks as proxies of the engagement of brain circuits that reflect resilience may help define prospective neurobehavioral markers of resilience. Such studies can reveal differences between resilient and stress-prone phenotypes and point out strategies by which stress-susceptible individuals could become more resilient. Vicentic emphasized that recent advances in computational modeling can rapidly test hypotheses about important features of resilience that would be difficult to address experimentally. By incorporating environmental, social, and neurophysiological variables important for resilience into different models, predictions about specific features of resilience can be tested. These approaches might reveal novel theoretical frameworks of resilience and illuminate factors that influence resilient responses to stress.

Frances Jensen expanded on the understanding of resilience as an adaptive phenomenon shaped by an evolving environment. She observed that in today's world—bombarded by digital media and unforeseen societal shifts—the brain's capacity for adaptability (or neuroplasticity) is continually challenged. Jensen introduced the concept of domain-specific resilience, suggesting that individuals may display resilience in certain aspects of life while remaining vulnerable in others. She elaborated on the promise of integrating molecular assessments such as transcriptomics, neuroendocrine markers, and behavioral indicators to detect subtle deficits in resilience before overt symptoms of toxic stress emerge. Recognizing the importance of a precision approach, Jensen emphasized aligning early biomarkers across multiple levels with targeted intervention strategies. She underscored the need for an expanded research agenda that integrates mechanistic, behavioral, and clinical dimensions to capture the prodromal signals of diminished resilience.

Reconceptualizing resilience as a biological trait, John Krystal offered a multifaceted view of resilience through the metaphor of a rock climber navigating perilous heights. A climber was shown ascending a risky route without a rope—Krystal delineated four aspects of resilience:

1. Low baseline stress activation: The climber maintains a steady composure even in high-stress situations.
2. Active coping: Despite facing dangerous conditions, the climber engages challenges dynamically.
3. Rebound capability: After moments of acute stress (illustrated by episodes of panic), the climber regains composure.
4. Traumatic growth: Post-adversity, the climber is propelled to take on even greater challenges.

Krystal introduced the provocative idea that if resilience is indeed a biological trait, then disruptions in the underlying mechanisms might be conceptualized as "diseases of resilience." He underscored findings from a meta-analysis of antidepressant trials that examined trajectories of response among thousands of patients to show that a subset of patients had responses even less favorable than placebo (Gueorguieva et al., 2011). This observation raised considerations about whether certain treatments may inadvertently compromise an individual's intrinsic capacity for resilience. He also referenced work by Peter Kramer, among others, to illustrate emerging evidence that some pharmacotherapies may operate not only by dampening symptoms but also by promoting a resilient epigenetic profile (Gueorguieva et al., 2011, 2017; Kramer, 1997; Krishnan et al., 2007; Nestler and Russo, 2024).

Husseini Manji built upon these themes by highlighting interventions that target the circuitry underlying stress responses. He noted that emerging data regarding AMPA (α-Amino-3-hydroxy-5-methyl-4-isoxazolepropionic acid)–mediated plasticity, which facilitates synaptic communication, suggest that pretreatment with NMDA antagonists (agents that modulate glutamate signaling) may protect against behavioral deficits induced by stress. Manji highlighted studies from Columbia University and Mount Sinai in which researchers demonstrated that interventions such as ketamine not only alleviate symptoms acutely but may also trigger adaptive processes within brain circuits. In discussing pharmacological agents, he mentioned that lithium—long valued for its mood-stabilizing properties—has been observed to reduce the duration of manic and depressive episodes and is linked to lower suicide rates (Kessing et al., 2005; Lewitzka et al., 2015; Sarai et al., 2018; Tondo and Baldessarini, 2024). These observations point to a dual role for some medications: both reducing immediate distress and potentially reinforcing resilience mechanisms by turning on resilience-promoting molecules like BAG1 (which regulates glucocorticoid receptor trafficking).

CHALLENGES AFTER STRESS RECOVERY

Jon Nelson shared a personal narrative that illustrated the complexities of stress recovery. He recounted the challenges of shifting from a state marked by overwhelming fatigue and depressive inertia to one where he must relearn how to feel and respond to emotional triggers. He even observed his children's responses to environmental cues (e.g., the sound of a barking dog or Nelson taking a nap) to anticipate his behavior before his recovery. These cues still trigger a stress response in his children today. Nelson emphasized that even after his recovery from a disease state, for him and his family, adapting to everyday stressors is a continual process, revealing the real-world implications of building resilience intergenerationally.

Nelson also reflected on a pivotal conversation with his doctor, Helen Mayberg, that helped him understand that his inability to engage in daily activities was due to abulia, a neurological impairment affecting motivation. While this revelation was validating, it also raised new concerns for him. Despite knowing that exercise and other healthy habits would improve his well-being, Nelson found himself unable to engage in them. Nelson wondered whether a form of behavioral abulia might persist even after recovery, making it difficult to fully reintegrate into daily life.

DISCUSSION

The Impact of the Digital Era

The potential of communication tools to extend education on stress and resilience across the lifespan was a recurring theme during the discussion. Jensen remarked that our modern environment inundates us with "terabytes of information" through digital media—a factor that, on one hand, can tax the brain's adaptive capacities yet, on the other, offers an opportunity. One online participant suggested that the formation of new social networks, driven by digital connectivity, might provide essential support for students leaving familiar environments and could help foster resilience in academic and professional settings.

The Importance of Interdisciplinary Collaboration and Research

Deanna Barch discussed a critical gap that remains in the measurement of resilience. She pointed to Nadine Burke Harris's earlier statement that research efforts are often siloed, with different studies focusing either on molecular markers or on clinical and behavioral assessments. By championing multidisciplinary projects that evaluate stress responses from the cellular to the societal level, researchers may better capture the multidimensional nature of resilience. For instance, Herman Taylor discussed some investigations in cardiovascular research that have employed pragmatic measures such as Life's Simple 7[1] to serve as proxies for resilience in primary care settings (Taylor et al., 2022). These integrative approaches underscore the possibility that clarity on resilience measurement will emerge only when diverse perspectives converge.

Burke Harris provided a detailed perspective on resilience measures, explaining how her team, both in clinical work and the surgeon general's office, has focused on regulating the physiologic stress response and addressing neuroendocrine immune and genetic disruptions. She highlighted the importance of examining resilience across different levels—molecular, physiologic, clinical, and community—and emphasized the need to connect basic science research with practical applications in primary care. Burke Harris advocated for measures that support early detection and intervention, noting

[1] Life's Simple 7, as defined by the American Heart Association, outlines seven key metrics for ideal cardiovascular health: maintaining a nonsmoking status, a body mass index below 25 kg/m^2, adherence to a heart-healthy diet, engaging in at least 150 minutes of moderate physical activity per week, keeping total blood cholesterol under 200 mg/dL, maintaining blood pressure below 120/80 mmHg, and ensuring fasting blood glucose remains under 100 mg/dL (Diaz-Gutierrez et al., 2023).

that California's precision medicine investments aim to identify therapeutic targets for toxic stress. She emphasized the importance of aligning research approaches with intended therapeutic goals, pointing to stem cell research as a model. Burke Harris stated that California funds these initiatives to advance the discovery of new treatments, demonstrating how a research framework can be strategically designed to develop therapeutic targets. She proposed that a similar approach could be applied to toxic stress, ensuring interventions address its underlying biological mechanisms rather than just its symptoms.

Opportunities for Intervention

A workshop participant emphasized that workplace stress is increasingly linked to declines in employee well-being and productivity. The participant called for greater research attention on resilience in professional settings, highlighting the critical role workplaces play within every community.

The discussion also explored cognitive behavioral therapy (CBT) as a tool for reprogramming thought patterns—an approach metaphorically likened to updating a space probe's software to fix hardware malfunctions. A workshop participant noted that, just as NASA finds ways to work around technical limitations, CBT helps individuals adapt by restructuring their cognitive responses to psychological challenges. Nestler added that this underscores the idea that resilience is not merely an inherent trait but a skill that can be taught.

Looking Forward

By interweaving insights from basic biological research, clinical practice, and public health communication, the discussions captured in this session offer a multifaceted view of resilience. Workshop participants reflected on the opportunities ahead to identify early biological markers, advance clinical interventions that not only alleviate symptoms but also strengthen innate adaptive mechanisms, and harness digital and social media to expand these strategies within communities.

CONCLUDING REMARKS

In reflecting on the workshop's discussions, there is growing recognition that the understanding of resilience is evolving into a more nuanced picture—one that goes beyond simply mitigating stress (for key points raised throughout the workshop, see Box 7-1). As Huda Akil explained, "It's like we've been studying microbes, but we don't know about antibodies," a metaphor that challenged the audience to not only investigate the threats individuals might

BOX 7-1
Key Points Raised Throughout the Workshop by Individual Speakers

- Researchers emphasized the importance of refining methods for translating findings across species and shifting from a trauma-informed approach to resilience-building, considering factors like timing of stress exposure and mechanisms for positive adaptation. Even reverse translation, taking results from human studies and studying them in preclinical models, can be a powerful approach for identifying therapeutic targets. (Baratta, Cameron, Dias, Kheirbek, Peña)
- Identifying reproducible biomarkers, molecular targets, and neural circuits can allow for more objective and biologically grounded diagnoses and resilience-building interventions that could have lasting generational effects. (Jensen, Manji, Ressler, Russo, Saxbe)
- There remain challenges in defining resilience, especially across animal models, disorders, and life stage. (Hyde, Ressler, Vicentic)
- Resilience happens dynamically over the lifespan, from infancy to adulthood. Systemic and social support are critical to the development and maintenance of resilience. (Akil, Birto, Hyde, Minnis, Nelson, Nestler)
- Chronic adversity does not just increase susceptibility to mental health challenges—it interacts dynamically with biological development, and environmental exposures over time impact multiple body systems like the microbiome and cardiovascular and immune systems. (Bremner, Burke Harris, Gur, Krystal, Montalvo-Ortiz)
- Public health interventions, such as childhood cognitive flexibility training, prenatal emotional regulation programs, stress management apps, and structured sleep education programs, could foster resilience on a population level and improve long-term well-being. (Burke Harris, Cameron, McBride Murry, Meaney, Rogers)
- Early intervention, childhood adversity, and systemic resilience-building could be positioned as public health priorities with nationwide implications. (Burke Harris, McBride Murry)

face but to also learn more about the mechanisms that could protect them. Her remarks on measuring stress fitness to help gauge whether an individual's stress levels are facilitating adaptation or signaling wear—whether through stress biomarkers, cardiovascular response, sleep tracking, or learned coping mechanisms—underscore a key area still ripe for inquiry. The conversation raised an important question about how to accurately measure resilience.

Akil's concept of an "emotional algebra" further anchored this discussion, suggesting that resilience is built on the calibrated mix of negative and positive experiences. By framing stress as both a challenge and a resource, she encouraged the consideration of different coping strategies across both individuals and communities, without casting any one approach as superior. Akil remarked that while the dialogue has sharpened the focus on these ideas, this also presents open questions about how best to integrate these measures into practical frameworks. Akil emphasized that the wisdom shared by those with lived experience is not only valuable but essential—shaping physiological, psychological, medical, and economic outcomes. She urged the scientific community to embrace and advocate for resilience as a legitimate field of study, underscoring its profound impact and its transformative potential for the greater good.

Appendix A

References

Akil, H., and E. J. Nestler. 2023. The neurobiology of stress: Vulnerability, resilience, and major depression. *Proceedings of the National Academy of Sciences* 120(49):e2312662120.

Aoued, H. S., S. Sannigrahi, N. Doshi, F. G. Morrison, H. Linsenbaum, S. C. Hunter, H. Walum, J. Baman, B. Yao, P. Jin, K. J. Ressler, and B. G. Dias. 2019. Reversing behavioral, neuroanatomical, and germline influences of intergenerational stress. *Biological Psychiatry* 85(3):248–256.

Aurbach, E. L., E. G. Inui, C. A. Turner, M. H. Hagenauer, K. E. Prater, J. Z. Li, D. Absher, N. Shah, P. Blandino, Jr., W. E. Bunney, R. M. Myers, J. D. Barchas, A. F. Schatzberg, S. J. Watson, Jr., and H. Akil. 2015. Fibroblast growth factor 9 is a novel modulator of negative affect. *Proceedings of the National Academy of Sciences* 112(38):11953–11958.

Baratta, M. V., N. R. Leslie, I. P. Fallon, S. D. Dolzani, L. E. Chun, A. M. Tamalunas, L. R. Watkins, and S. F. Maier. 2018. Behavioural and neural sequelae of stressor exposure are not modulated by controllability in females. *European Journal of Neuroscience* 47(8):959–967.

Bennett, S. N., A. B. Chang, F. D. Rogers, P. Jones, and C. J. Peña. 2024. Thyroid hormones mediate the impact of early-life stress on ventral tegmental area gene expression and behavior. *Hormones and Behavior* 159:105472.

Bick, J., T. Zhu, C. Stamoulis, N. A. Fox, C. Zeanah, and C. A. Nelson. 2015. Effect of early institutionalization and foster care on long-term white matter development: A randomized clinical trial. *JAMA Pediatrics* 169(3):211–219.

Brady, R. G., C. E. Rogers, T. Prochaska, S. Kaplan, R. E. Lean, T. A. Smyser, J. S. Shimony, G. M. Slavich, B. B. Warner, D. M. Barch, J. L. Luby, and C. D. Smyser. 2022. The effects of prenatal exposure to neighborhood crime on neonatal functional connectivity. *Biological Psychiatry* 92(2):139–148.

Bremner, J. D., N. Z. Gurel, Y. Jiao, M. T. Wittbrodt, O. M. Levantsevych, M. Huang, H. Jung, M. H. Shandhi, J. Beckwith, I. Herring, M. H. Rapaport, N. Murrah, E. Driggers, Y. A. Ko, M. L. Alkhalaf, M. Soudan, J. Song, B. S. Ku, L. Shallenberger, A. N. Hankus, J. A. Nye, J. Park, V. Vaccarino, A. J. Shah, O. T. Inan, and B. D. Pearce. 2020. Transcutaneous vagal nerve stimulation blocks stress-induced activation of interleukin-6 and interferon-gamma in posttraumatic stress disorder: A double-blind, randomized, sham-controlled trial. *Brain, Behavior, and Immunity—Health* 9:100138.

Brody, G.H., T. Yu, Y. F. Chen, S. M. Kogan, G. W. Evans, S. R. Beach, M. Windle, R. L. Simons, M. Gerrard, F. X. Gibbons, and R. A. Philibert. 2013. Cumulative socioeconomic status risk, allostatic load, and adjustment: A prospective latent profile analysis with contextual and genetic protective factors. *Developmental Psychology* 49(5):913–927.

California First 5. 2025. *What We Do*. https://www.ccfc.ca.gov/whatwedo/index.html (accessed June 4, 2025).

Cameron, J. L., K. L. Eagleson, N. A. Fox, T. K. Hensch, and P. Levitt. 2017. Social origins of developmental risk for mental and physical illness. *Journal of Neuroscience* 37(45):10783–10791.

Campbell-Sills, L., S. B. Norman, M. G. Craske, G. Sullivan, A. J. Lang, D. A. Chavira, A. Bystritsky, C. Sherbourne, P. Roy-Byrne, and M. B. Stein. 2009. Validation of a brief measure of anxiety-related severity and impairment: The Overall Anxiety Severity and Impairment Scale (OASIS). *Journal of Affective Disorders* 112(1–3):92–101.

Cardenas, S. I., Y. Waizman, V. Truong, P. Sellery, S. A. Stoycos, F. C. Yeh, V. Rajagopalan, and D. E. Saxbe. 2024. White matter microstructure organization across the transition to fatherhood. *Developmental Cognitive Neuroscience* 67:101374.

Carmona, S. 2024. *Neuromaternal: ¿Qué Le Pasa a Mi Cerebro Durante El Embarazo Y La Maternidad?* PRH Grupo Editorial.

Chino, M., and L. Debruyn. 2006. Building true capacity: Indigenous models for Indigenous communities. *American Journal of Public Health* 96(4):596–599.

Conger, R. D., K. J. Conger, G. H. Elder, Jr., F. O. Lorenz, R. L. Simons, and L. B. Whitbeck. 1992. A family process model of economic hardship and adjustment of early adolescent boys. *Child Development* 63(3):526–541.

COVID-19 Mental Disorders Collaborators. 2021. Global prevalence and burden of depressive and anxiety disorders in 204 countries and territories in 2020 due to the COVID-19 pandemic. *Lancet* 398(10312):1700–1712.

Del Giudice, M., B. J. Ellis, and E. A. Shirtcliff. 2011. The Adaptive Calibration Model of Stress Responsivity. *Neuroscience and Biobehavioral Reviews* 35(7):1562–1592.

Dias, B. G., and K. J. Ressler. 2014. Parental olfactory experience influences behavior and neural structure in subsequent generations. *Nature Neuroscience* 17(1):89–96.

Diaz-Gutierrez, J., M. A. Martinez-Gonzalez, A. Alonso, E. Toledo, J. Salas-Salvado, J. V. Sorli, E. Ros, M. Fito, R. Estruch, F. Aros, M. Fiol, J. Lapetra, E. Gomez-Gracia, L. Serra-Majem, X. Pinto, O. Portoles, N. Babio, O. Castaner, and M. Ruiz-Canela. 2023. American Heart Association's Life Simple 7 and the risk of atrial fibrillation in the PREDIMED study cohort. *Nutrition, Metabolism and Cardiovascular Diseases* 33(6):1144–1148.

Evans, S. J., P. V. Choudary, C. R. Neal, J. Z. Li, M. P. Vawter, H. Tomita, J. F. Lopez, R. C. Thompson, F. Meng, J. D. Stead, D. M. Walsh, R. M. Myers, W. E. Bunney, S. J. Watson, E. G. Jones, and H. Akil. 2004. Dysregulation of the fibroblast growth factor system in major depression. *Proceedings of the National Academy of Sciences* 101(43):15506–15511.

Felitti, V. J., R. F. Anda, D. Nordenberg, D. F. Williamson, A. M. Spitz, V. Edwards, and J. S. Marks. 1998. Relationship of childhood abuse and household dysfunction to many of the leading causes of death in adults: The Adverse Childhood Experiences (ACE) Study. *American Journal of Preventive Medicine* 14(4):245–258.

Fernandes, G., M. Fernandes, N. Vaidya, P. De Souza, E. Plotnikova, R. Geddes, B. Holla, E. Sharma, V. Benegal, and V. Choudhry. 2021. Prevalence of child maltreatment in India and its association with gender, urbanisation and policy: A rapid review and meta-analysis protocol. *BMJ Open* 11(8):e044983.

Galley, J. D., M. K. King, T. A. Rajasekera, A. Batabyal, S. T. Woodke, and T. L. Gur. 2024. Gestational administration of bifidobacterium dentium results in intergenerational modulation of inflammatory, metabolic, and social behavior. *Brain, Behavior, and Immunity—Health* 122:44–57.

Galley, J. D., L. Mashburn-Warren, L. C. Blalock, C. L. Lauber, J. E. Carroll, K. M. Ross, C. Hobel, M. Coussons-Read, C. Dunkel Schetter, and T. L. Gur. 2023. Maternal anxiety, depression and stress affects offspring gut microbiome diversity and bifidobacterial abundances. *Brain, Behavior, and Immunity—Health* 107:253–264.

Gard, A. M., J. Brooks-Gunn, S. S. McLanahan, C. Mitchell, C. S. Monk, and L. W. Hyde. 2022a. Deadly gun violence, neighborhood collective efficacy, and adolescent neurobehavioral outcomes. *PNAS Nexus* 1(3):pgac061.

Gard, A. M., T. C. Hein, C. Mitchell, J. Brooks-Gunn, S. S. McLanahan, C. S. Monk, and L. W. Hyde. 2022b. Prospective longitudinal associations between harsh parenting and corticolimbic function during adolescence. *Development and Psychopathology* 34(3):981–996.

Gard, A. M., R. Waller, D. S. Shaw, E. E. Forbes, A. R. Hariri, and L. W. Hyde. 2017. The long reach of early adversity: Parenting, stress, and neural pathways to antisocial behavior in adulthood. *Biological Psychiatry: Cognitive Neuroscience and Neuroimaging* 2(7):582–590.

Geiger, L. T., J. R. Balouek, M. R. Barrett, J. M. Thompson, L. Z. Fang, L. A. Farrelly, A. S. Chen, M. Tang, S. N. Bennett, B. A. Garcia, I. Maze, M. C. Creed, and C. J. Peña. 2025. Early-life stress alters chromatin modifications in VTA to prime stress sensitivity. *bioRxiv*.

Gillespie, M. L., A. Sharma, T. G. M. Van Erp, M. Ernst, V. M. Murry, and U. Rao. 2020. Functional connectivity during reward-seeking in adolescents enrolled in a risk-reduction intervention. *Society of Biological Psychiatry Annual Meeting*.

Gueorguieva, R., A. M. Chekroud, and J. H. Krystal. 2017. Trajectories of relapse in randomised, placebo-controlled trials of treatment discontinuation in major depressive disorder: An individual patient-level data meta-analysis. *Lancet Psychiatry* 4(3):230–237.

Gueorguieva, R., C. Mallinckrodt, and J. H. Krystal. 2011. Trajectories of depression severity in clinical trials of duloxetine: Insights into antidepressant and placebo responses. *Archives of General Psychiatry* 68(12):1227–1237.

Gumusoglu, S. B. 2024. The role of the placenta-brain axis in psychoneuroimmune programming. *Brain, Behavior, and Immunity—Health* 36:100735.

Gur, T. L., A. V. Palkar, T. Rajasekera, J. Allen, A. Niraula, J. Godbout, and M. T. Bailey. 2019. Prenatal stress disrupts social behavior, cortical neurobiology and commensal microbes in adult male offspring. *Behavioral Brain Research* 359:886–894.

Gur, T. L., L. Shay, A. V. Palkar, S. Fisher, V. A. Varaljay, S. Dowd, and M. T. Bailey. 2017. Prenatal stress affects placental cytokines and neurotrophins, commensal microbes, and anxiety-like behavior in adult female offspring. *Brain, Behavior, and Immunity—Health* 64:50–58.

Herry, C., S. Ciocchi, V. Senn, L. Demmou, C. Muller, and A. Lüthi. 2008. Switching on and off fear by distinct neuronal circuits. *Nature* 454(7204):600–606.

Hiller, R. M., S. Lehmann, S. J. Lewis, H. Minnis, K. H. Shelton, M. Tarren-Sweeney, and H. N. Taussig. 2023. Accommodating complexity: The need for evidence-informed mental health assessments for children in out-of-home care. *Journal of the American Academy of Child and Adolescent Psychiatry* 62(1):12–18.

Ho, T. C., and L. S. King. 2021. Mechanisms of neuroplasticity linking early adversity to depression: Developmental considerations. *Translational Psychiatry* 11(1):517.

Hoekzema, E., E. Barba-Muller, C. Pozzobon, M. Picado, F. Lucco, D. Garcia-Garcia, J. C. Soliva, A. Tobena, M. Desco, E. A. Crone, A. Ballesteros, S. Carmona, and O. Vilarroya. 2017. Pregnancy leads to long-lasting changes in human brain structure. *Nature Neuroscience* 20(2):287–296.

Hyde, L. W., A. M. Gard, R. C. Tomlinson, G. L. Suarez and H. B. Westerman. 2022. Parents, neighborhoods, and the developing brain. *Child Development Perspectives* 16:148-156.

Hyde, L. W., R. Waller, C. J. Trentacosta, D. S. Shaw, J. M. Neiderhiser, J. M. Ganiban, D. Reiss, and L. D. Leve. 2016. Heritable and nonheritable pathways to early callous-unemotional behaviors. *American Journal of Psychiatry* 173(9):903–910.

Jones, S. V., L. Stanek-Rattiner, M. Davis, and K. J. Ressler. 2007. Differential regional expression of brain-derived neurotrophic factor following olfactory fear learning. *Learning and Memory* 14(12):816–820.

Jovanovic, T., A. Smith, A. Kamkwalala, J. Poole, T. Samples, S. D. Norrholm, K. J. Ressler, and B. Bradley. 2011. Physiological markers of anxiety are increased in children of abused mothers. *Journal of Child Psychology and Psychiatry and Allied Disciplines*, 52(8):844–852.

Katrinli, S., A. X. Maihofer, A. H. Wani, J. R. Pfeiffer, E. Ketema, A. Ratanatharathorn, D. G. Baker, M. P. Boks, E. Geuze, R. C. Kessler, V. B. Risbrough, B. P. F. Rutten, M. B. Stein, R. J. Ursano, E. Vermetten, M. W. Logue, C. M. Nievergelt, A. K. Smith, and M. Uddin. 2022. Epigenome-wide meta-analysis of PTSD symptom severity in three military cohorts implicates DNA methylation changes in genes involved in immune system and oxidative stress. *Molecular Psychiatry* 27(3):1720–1728.

Kaufman, J., J. L. Montalvo-Ortiz, H. Holbrook, K. O'Loughlin, C. Orr, C. Kearney, B. Z. Yang, T. Wang, H. Zhao, R. Althoff, H. Garavan, J. Gelernter, and J. Hudziak. 2018. Adverse childhood experiences, epigenetic measures, and obesity in youth. *Journal of Pediatrics* 202:150–156.

Kee, M. Z. L., A. Cremaschi, M. De Iorio, H. Chen, T. Montreuil, T. V. Nguyen, S. M. Cote, K. J. O'Donnell, G. F. Giesbrecht, N. Letourneau, S. Y. Chan, and M. J. Meaney. 2023. Perinatal trajectories of maternal depressive symptoms in prospective, community-based cohorts across 3 continents. *JAMA Network Open* 6(10):e2339942.

Kessing, L. V., L. Sondergard, K. Kvist, and P. K. Andersen. 2005. Suicide risk in patients treated with lithium. *Archives of General Psychiatry* 62(8):860–866.

Kochanek, K. D., S. L. Murphy, J. Xu, and E. Arias. 2022. *Mortality in the United States.* National Center for Health Statistics.

Kramer, P. D. 1997. *Listening to Prozac: The Landmark Book About Antidepressants and the Remaking of the Self.* Penguin Life.

Krishnan, V., M. H. Han, D. L. Graham, O. Berton, W. Renthal, S. J. Russo, Q. Laplant, A. Graham, M. Lutter, D. C. Lagace, S. Ghose, R. Reister, P. Tannous, T. A. Green, R. L. Neve, S. Chakravarty, A. Kumar, A. J. Eisch, D. W. Self, F. S. Lee, C. A. Tamminga, D. C. Cooper, H. K. Gershenfeld, and E. J. Nestler. 2007. Molecular adaptations underlying susceptibility and resistance to social defeat in brain reward regions. *Cell* 131(2):391–404.

Lei, M. K., M. T. Berg, R. L. Simons, and S. R. H. Beach. 2022. Neighborhood structural disadvantage and biological aging in a sample of Black middle age and young adults. *Social Science and Medicine* 293:114654.

Leverett, S. D., R. G. Brady, U. A. Tooley, R. E. Lean, R. Tillman, J. Wilson, M. Ruscitti, R. L. Triplett, D. Alexopoulos, E. D. Gerstein, T. A. Smyser, B. Warner, J. L. Luby, C. D. Smyser, C. E. Rogers, and D. M. Barch. 2025. Associations between parenting and cognitive and language abilities at 2 years of age depend on prenatal exposure to disadvantage. *Journal of Pediatrics* 276:114289.

Lewitzka, U., E. Severus, R. Bauer, P. Ritter, B. Muller-Oerlinghausen, and M. Bauer. 2015. The suicide prevention effect of lithium: More than 20 years of evidence—A narrative review. *International Journal of Bipolar Disorders* 3(1):32.

Li, L., R. Durand-de Cuttoli, A. V. Aubry, C. J. Burnett, F. Cathomas, L. F. Parise, K. L. Chan, C. Morel, C. Yuan, Y. Shimo, H. Y. Lin, J. Wang, and S. J. Russo. 2023. Social trauma engages lateral septum circuitry to occlude social reward. *Nature* 613(7945):696–703.

Luby, J. L., M. P. Herzberg, C. Hoyniak, R. Tillman, R. E. Lean, R. Brady, R. Triplett, D. Alexopoulos, D. Loseille, T. Smyser, C. E. Rogers, B. Warner, C. D. Smyser, and D. M. Barch. 2024. Basic environmental supports for positive brain and cognitive development in the first year of life. *JAMA Pediatrics* 178(5):465–472.

Lutz, P. E., A. Tanti, A. Gasecka, S. Barnett-Burns, J. J. Kim, Y. Zhou, G. G. Chen, M. Wakid, M. Shaw, D. Almeida, M. A. Chay, J. Yang, V. Lariviere, M. N. M'Boutchou, L. C. van Kempen, V. Yerko, J. Prud'homme, M. A. Davoli, K. Vaillancourt, J. F. Theroux, A. Bramoulle, T. Y. Zhang, M. J. Meaney, C. Ernst, D. Cote, N. Mechawar, and G. Turecki. 2017. Association of a history of child abuse with impaired myelination in the anterior cingulate cortex: Convergent epigenetic, transcriptional, and morphological evidence. *American Journal of Psychiatry* 174(12):1185–1194.

Maier, S. F., and L. R. Watkins. 2005. Stressor controllability and learned helplessness: The roles of the dorsal raphe nucleus, serotonin, and corticotropin-releasing factor. *Neuroscience and Biobehavioral Reviews* 29(4–5):829–841.

Makino, Y., N. W. Hodgson, E. Doenier, A. V. Serbin, K. Osada, P. Artoni, M. Dickey, B. Sullivan, A. Potter-Dickey, J. Komanchuk, B. Sekhon, N. Letourneau, N. D. Ryan, J. Trauth, J. L. Cameron, and T. K. Hensch. 2024. Sleep-sensitive dopamine receptor expression in male mice underlies attention deficits after a critical period of early adversity. *Science Translational Medicine* 16(768):eadh9763.

Martinez-Garcia, M., M. Paternina-Die, S. I. Cardenas, O. Vilarroya, M. Desco, S. Carmona, and D. E. Saxbe. 2023. First-time fathers show longitudinal gray matter cortical volume reductions: Evidence from two international samples. *Cerebral Cortex* 33(7):4156–4163.

McEwen, B. S., and H. Akil. 2020. Revisiting the stress concept: Implications for affective disorders. *Journal of Neuroscience* 40(1):12–21.

Menard, C., and S. J. Russo. 2018. Non-invasive chemogenetics. *Nature Biomedical Engineering* 2(7):467–468.

Merrick, M.T., D. C. Ford, K. A. Ports, A. S. Guinn, J. Chen, J. Klevens, M. Metzler, C. M. Jones, T. R. Simon, V. M. Daniel, P. Ottley, and J. A. Mercy. 2019. Vital signs: Estimated proportion of adult health problems attributable to adverse childhood experiences and implications for prevention—25 states, 2015–2017. *MMWR. Morbidity and Mortality Weekly Report* 68(44):999–1005.

Miller, G. E., G. H. Brody, T. Yu, and E. Chen. 2014. A family-oriented psychosocial intervention reduces inflammation in low-SES African American youth. *Proceedings of the National Academy of Sciences* 111(31):11287–11292.

Miller-Graff, L. E. 2022. The multidimensional taxonomy of individual resilience. *Trauma, Violence, and Abuse* 23(2):660–675.

Minnis, H. 2013. Maltreatment-associated psychiatric problems: An example of environmentally triggered essence? *Scientific World Journal* 2013:148468.

Minnis, H., A.-L. van Harmelen, R. Gajwani, J. Rizeq, E. Combet, R. M. Reynolds, C. Gillberg, M. Henderson, F. K. Ho, V. Mondelli, J. Pell, J. Smith, and P. G. Shiels. 2024. The bio-exposome: Intracellular processes, stress physiology and the environment. *Nature Mental Health* 2:132–140.

Moazzami, K., M. T. Wittbrodt, M. Alkhalaf, B. B. Lima, J. A. Nye, P. K. Mehta, A. A. Quyyumi, V. Vaccarino, J. D. Bremner, and A. J. Shah. 2020. Association between mental stress-induced inferior frontal cortex activation and angina in coronary artery disease. *Circulation: Cardiovascular Imaging* 13(8):e010710.

Montalvo-Ortiz, J. L., J. Gelernter, Z. Cheng, M. J. Girgenti, K. Xu, X. Zhang, S. Gopalan, H. Zhou, R. S. Duman, S. M. Southwick, J. H. Krystal, G. Traumatic Stress Brain Research Study, and R. H. Pietrzak. 2022. Epigenome-wide association study of posttraumatic stress disorder identifies novel loci in U.S. military veterans. *Translational Psychiatry* 12(1):65.

Morgan, C. A., III, S. Wang, S. M. Southwick, A. Rasmusson, G. Hazlett, R. L. Hauger, and D. S. Charney. 2000. Plasma neuropeptide-Y concentrations in humans exposed to military survival training. *Biological Psychiatry* 47(10):902–909.

Morrison, F. G., B. G. Dias, and K. J. Ressler. 2015. Extinction reverses olfactory fear-conditioned increases in neuron number and glomerular size. *Proceedings of the National Academy of Sciences* 112(41):12846–12851.

Murry, V. M., J. M. Nyanamba, R. Hanebutt, M. Debreaux, K. A. B. Gastineau, A. K. B. Goodwin, and L. Narisetti. 2023. Critical examination of resilience and resistance in African American families: Adaptive capacities to navigate toxic oppressive upstream waters. *Development and Psychopathology* 35(5):2113–2131.

Navarrete, J., K. N. Schneider, B. M. Smith, N. L. Goodwin, Y. Y. Zhang, A. S. Salazar, Y. E. Gonzalez, P. Anumolu, E. Gross, V. S. Tsai, M. Heshmati, and S. A. Golden. 2024. Individual differences in volitional social self-administration and motivation in male and female mice following social stress. *Biological Psychiatry* 96(4):309–321.

Nestler, E. J., and S. J. Russo. 2024. Neurobiological basis of stress resilience. *Neuron* 112(12):1911–1929.

Nievergelt, C. M., A. X. Maihofer, E. G. Atkinson, C. Y. Chen, K. W. Choi, J. R. I. Coleman, N. P. Daskalakis, L. E. Duncan, R. Polimanti, C. Aaronson, A. B. Amstadter, S. B. Andersen, O. A. Andreassen, P. A. Arbisi, A. E. Ashley-Koch, S. B. Austin, E. Avdibegovic, D. Babic, S. A. Bacanu, D. G. Baker, A. Batzler, J. C. Beckham, S. Belangero, C. Benjet, C. Bergner, L. M. Bierer, J. M. Biernacka, L. J. Bierut, J. I. Bisson, M. P. Boks, E. A. Bolger, A. Brandolino, G. Breen, R. A. Bressan, R. A. Bryant, A. C. Bustamante, J. Bybjerg-Grauholm, M. Baekvad-Hansen, A. D. Borglum, S. Borte, L. Cahn, J. R. Calabrese, J. M. Caldas-de-Almeida, C. Chatzinakos, S. Cheema, S. A. P. Clouston, L. Colodro-Conde, B. J. Coombes, C. S. Cruz-Fuentes, A. M. Dale, S. Dalvie, L. K. Davis, J. Deckert, D. L. Delahanty, M. F. Dennis, F. Desarnaud, C. P. DiPietro, S. G. Disner, A. R. Docherty, K. Domschke, G. Dyb, A. D. Kulenovic, H. J. Edenberg, A. Evans, C. Fabbri, N. Fani, L. A. Farrer, A. Feder, N. C. Feeny, J. D. Flory, D. Forbes, C. E. Franz, S. Galea, M. E. Garrett, B. Gelaye, J. Gelernter, E. Geuze, C. F. Gillespie, S. B. Goleva, S. D. Gordon, A. Goci, L. R. Grasser, C. Guindalini, M. Haas, S. Hagenaars, M. A. Hauser, A. C. Heath, S. M. J. Hemmings, V. Hesselbrock, I. B. Hickie, K. Hogan, D. M. Hougaard, H. Huang, L. M. Huckins, K. Hveem, M. Jakovljevic, A. Javanbakht, G. D. Jenkins, J. Johnson, I. Jones, T. Jovanovic, K. I. Karstoft, M. L. Kaufman, J. L. Kennedy, R. C. Kessler, A. Khan, N. A. Kimbrel, A. P. King, N. Koen, R. Kotov, H. R. Kranzler, K. Krebs, W. S. Kremen, P. F. Kuan, B. R. Lawford, L. A. M. Lebois, K. Lehto, D. F. Levey, C. Lewis, I. Liberzon, S. D. Linnstaedt, M. W. Logue, A. Lori, Y. Lu, B. J. Luft, M. K. Lupton, J. J. Luykx, I. Makotkine, J. L. Maples-Keller, S. Marchese, C. Marmar, N. G. Martin, G. A. Martinez-Levy, K. McAloney, A. McFarlane, K. A. McLaughlin, S. A. McLean, S. E. Medland, D. Mehta, J. Meyers, V. Michopoulos, E. A. Mikita, L. Milani, W. Milberg, M. W. Miller, R. A. Morey, C. P. Morris, O. Mors, P. B. Mortensen, M. S. Mufford, E. C. Nelson, M. Nordentoft, S. B. Norman, N. R. Nugent, M. O'Donnell, H. K. Orcutt, P. M. Pan, M. S. Panizzon, G. A. Pathak, E. S. Peters, A. L. Peterson, M. Peverill, R. H. Pietrzak, M. A. Polusny, B. Porjesz, A. Powers, X. J. Qin, A. Ratanatharathorn, V. B. Risbrough, A. L. Roberts, A. O. Rothbaum, B. O. Rothbaum, P. Roy-Byrne, K. J. Ruggiero, A. Rung, H. Runz, B. P. F. Rutten, S. S. de Viteri, G. A. Salum, L. Sampson, S. E. Sanchez, M. Santoro, C. Seah, S. Seedat, J. S. Seng, A. Shabalin, C. M. Sheerin, D. Silove, A. K. Smith, J. W. Smoller, S. R. Sponheim, D. J. Stein, S. Stensland, J. S. Stevens, J. A. Sumner, M. H. Teicher, W. K. Thompson, A. K. Tiwari, E. Trapido, M. Uddin, R. J. Ursano, U. Valdimarsdottir, M. Van Hooff, E. Vermetten, C. H. Vinkers, J. Voisey, Y. Wang, Z. Wang, M. Waszczuk, H. Weber, F. R. Wendt, T. Werge, M. A. Williams, D. E. Williamson, B. S. Winsvold, S. Winternitz, C. Wolf, E. J. Wolf, Y. Xia, Y. Xiong, R. Yehuda, K. A. Young, R. M. Young, C. C. Zai, G. C. Zai, M. Zervas, H. Zhao, L. A. Zoellner, J. A. Zwart, T. deRoon-Cassini, S. J. H. van Rooij, L. L. van den Heuvel, A. Study, T. Estonian Biobank Research, I. FinnGen, H. A.-I. Psychiatry, M. B. Stein, K. J. Ressler, and K. C. Koenen. 2024. Genome-wide association analyses identify 95 risk loci and provide insights into the neurobiology of post-traumatic stress disorder. *Nature Genetics* 56(5):792–808.

Nunez-Rios, D. L., J. J. Martinez-Magana, S. T. Nagamatsu, D. E. Andrade-Brito, D. A. Forero, C. A. Orozco-Castano, and J. L. Montalvo-Ortiz. 2022. Central and peripheral immune dysregulation in posttraumatic stress disorder: Convergent multi-omics evidence. *Biomedicines* 10(5):1107.

Office of the California Surgeon General. 2025. *Adverse Childhood Experiences (ACEs) and Toxic Stress.* https://osg.ca.gov/aces-toxic-stress/ (accessed June 4, 2025).

Parade, S. H., L. Huffhines, T. E. Daniels, L. R. Stroud, N. R. Nugent, and A. R. Tyrka. 2021. A systematic review of childhood maltreatment and DNA methylation: Candidate gene and epigenome-wide approaches. *Translational Psychiatry* 11(1):134.

Pataskar, A., J. Jung, P. Smialowski, F. Noack, F. Calegari, T. Straub, and V. K. Tiwari. 2016. NeuroD1 reprograms chromatin and transcription factor landscapes to induce the neuronal program. *EMBO Journal* 35(1):24–45.

Peña, C. J. 2025. Early-life stress sensitizes response to future stress: Evidence and mechanisms. *Neurobiology of Stress* 35:100716.

Peña, C. J., H. G. Kronman, D. M. Walker, H. M. Cates, R. C. Bagot, I. Purushothaman, O. Issler, Y. E. Loh, T. Leong, D. D. Kiraly, E. Goodman, R. L. Neve, L. Shen, and E. J. Nestler. 2017. Early life stress confers lifelong stress susceptibility in mice via ventral tegmental area OTX2. *Science* 356(6343):1185–1188.

Peña, C. J., M. Smith, A. Ramakrishnan, H. M. Cates, R. C. Bagot, H. G. Kronman, B. Patel, A. B. Chang, I. Purushothaman, J. Dudley, H. Morishita, L. Shen, and E. J. Nestler. 2019. Early life stress alters transcriptomic patterning across reward circuitry in male and female mice. *Nature Communications* 10(1):5098.

Peterson, C., M. V. Aslam, P. H. Niolon, S. Bacon, M. A. Bellis, J. A. Mercy, and C. Florence. 2023. Economic burden of health conditions associated with adverse childhood experiences among US adults. *JAMA Network Open* 6(12):e2346323.

Putnam, K. T., W. W. Harris, and F. W. Putnam. 2013. Synergistic childhood adversities and complex adult psychopathology. *Journal of Traumatic Stress* 26(4):435–442.

Rajasekera, T. A., J. D. Galley, A. R. Mackos, H. J. Chen, J. G. Mitchell, J. J. Kleinman, P. Cappelucci, L. Mashburn-Warren, C. L. Lauber, M. T. Bailey, and B. L. Worly. 2024. Stress and depression-associated shifts in gut microbiota: A pilot study of human pregnancy. *Brain, Behavior, and Immunity—Health* 36:100730.

Rakers, F., S. Rupprecht, M. Dreiling, C. Bergmeier, O. W. Witte, and M. Schwab. 2017. Transfer of maternal psychosocial stress to the fetus. *Neuroscience and Biobehavioral Reviews* 117:185-197.

Reinert, M., D. Fritze, and T. Nguyen. 2024. *The State of Mental Health in America, 2024.* Mental Health America.

Ressler, K. J., B. O. Rothbaum, L. Tannenbaum, P. Anderson, K. Graap, E. Zimand, L. Hodges, and M. Davis. 2004. Cognitive enhancers as adjuncts to psychotherapy: Use of D-cycloserine in phobic individuals to facilitate extinction of fear. *Archives of General Psychiatry* 61(11):1136–1144.

Rutter, M. 1985. Resilience in the face of adversity: Protective factors and resistance to psychiatric disorder. *The British Journal of Psychiatry* 147(6):598–611.

Saad, L. 2025. *Pandemic's Effects Linger in Americans' Health Ratings.* Gallup.

Sanders, A. F. P., B. Tirado, N. A. Seider, R. L. Triplett, R. E. Lean, J. J. Neil, J. P. Miller, R. Tillman, T. A. Smyser, D. M. Barch, J. L. Luby, C. E. Rogers, C. D. Smyser, B. B. Warner, E. Chen, and G. E. Miller. 2024. Prenatal exposure to maternal disadvantage-related inflammatory biomarkers: Associations with neonatal white matter microstructure. *Translational Psychiatry* 14(1):72.

Sarai, S. K., H. M. Mekala, and S. Lippmann. 2018. Lithium suicide prevention: A brief review and reminder. *Innovations in Clinical Neuroscience* 15(11–12):30–32.

Saxbe, D., and M. Martinez-Garcia. 2024. Cortical volume reductions in men transitioning to first-time fatherhood reflect both parenting engagement and mental health risk. *Cerebral Cortex* 34(4):bhae126.

Sheftall, A. H. 2023. The tragedy of Black youth suicide. Association of American Medical Colleges.

Smith, G. D., and S. Ebrahim. 2003. "Mendelian randomization": Can genetic epidemiology contribute to understanding environmental determinants of disease? *International Journal of Epidemiology* 32(1):1–22.

Solmi, M., G. Seitidis, D. Mavridis, C. U. Correll, E. Dragioti, S. Guimond, L. Tuominen, A. Dargel, A. F. Carvalho, M. Fornaro, M. Maes, F. Monaco, M. Song, J. Il Shin, and S. Cortese. 2023. Incidence, prevalence, and global burden of schizophrenia—Data, with critical appraisal, from the global burden of disease (GBD) 2019. *Molecular Psychiatry* 28(12):5319–5327.

Stenson, A. F., S. J. H. van Rooij, S. E. Carter, A. Powers, and T. Jovanovic. 2021. A legacy of fear: Physiological evidence for intergenerational effects of trauma exposure on fear and safety signal learning among African Americans. *Behavioural Brain Research* 402:113017.

Suarez, G. L., S. A. Burt, A. M. Gard, J. Burton, D. A. Clark, K. L. Klump, and L. W. Hyde. 2022. The impact of neighborhood disadvantage on amygdala reactivity: Pathways through neighborhood social processes. *Developmental Cognitive Neuroscience* 54:101061.

Suarez, G. L., S. A. Burt, A. M. Gard, K. L. Klump, and L. W. Hyde. 2024. Exposure to community violence as a mechanism linking neighborhood disadvantage to amygdala reactivity and the protective role of parental nurturance. *Developmental Psychology* 60(4):595–609.

Taylor, H. A., T. Finkel, Y. Gao, S. W. Ballinger, R. Campo, R. Chen, S. H. Chen, K. Davidson, M. L. Iruela-Arispe, C. Jaquish, N. K. LeBrasseur, M. C. Odden, G. J. Papanicolaou, M. Picard, P. Srinivas, O. Tjurmina, M. Wolz, and Z. S. Galis. 2022. Scientific opportunities in resilience research for cardiovascular health and wellness. Report from a National Heart, Lung, and Blood Institute workshop. *The FASEB Journal* 36(12):e22639.

Taylor, W. W., L. Korobkova, N. Bhinderwala, and B. G. Dias. 2025. Toward understanding and halting legacies of trauma. *Biological Psychiatry* 98(10):756–766.

Tondo, L., and R. J. Baldessarini. 2024. Prevention of suicidal behavior with lithium treatment in patients with recurrent mood disorders. *International Journal of Bipolar Disorders* 12(1):6.

Turner, C. A., H. Khalil, V. Murphy-Weinberg, M. H. Hagenauer, L. Gates, Y. Tang, L. Weinberg, R. Grysko, L. Floran-Garduno, T. Dokas, C. Samaniego, Z. Zhao, Y. Fang, S. Sen, J. F. Lopez, S. J. Watson, Jr., and H. Akil. 2023. The impact of COVID-19 on a college freshman sample reveals genetic and nongenetic forms of susceptibility and resilience to stress. *Proceedings of the National Academy of Sciences* 120(49):e2305779120.

Turner, C. A., S. J. Watson, and H. Akil. 2012. The fibroblast growth factor family: Neuromodulation of affective behavior. *Neuron* 76(1):160–174.

Vaccarino, V., Z. Almuwaqqat, J. H. Kim, M. Hammadah, A. J. Shah, Y. A. Ko, L. Elon, S. Sullivan, A. Shah, A. Alkhoder, B. B. Lima, B. Pearce, L. Ward, M. Kutner, Y. Hu, T. T. Lewis, E. V. Garcia, J. Nye, D. S. Sheps, P. Raggi, J. D. Bremner, and A. A. Quyyumi. 2021. Association of mental stress-induced myocardial ischemia with cardiovascular events in patients with coronary heart disease. *JAMA* 326(18):1818–1828.

Vaccarino, V., J. Goldberg, C. Rooks, A. J. Shah, E. Veledar, T. L. Faber, J. R. Votaw, C. W. Forsberg, and J. D. Bremner. 2013. Post-traumatic stress disorder and incidence of coronary heart disease: A twin study. *Journal of the American College of Cardiology* 62(11):970–978.

Vaccarino, V., A. J. Shah, V. Moncayo, J. Nye, M. Piccinelli, Y. A. Ko, X. Ma, N. Murrah, L. Shallenberger, E. Driggers, O. M. Levantsevych, M. Hammadah, B. B. Lima, A. Young, W. O'Neal, M. Alkhalaf, A. Haffar, P. Raggi, J. Goldberg, N. L. Smith, E. V. Garcia, A. A. Quyyumi, and J. D. Bremner. 2022. Posttraumatic stress disorder, myocardial perfusion, and myocardial blood flow: A longitudinal twin study. *Biological Psychiatry* 91(7):615–625.

Verosky, B. G., M. T. Bailey, and T. L. Gur. 2025. The metabolomic mind: Microbial metabolite programming of microglia. *Neuroimmunomodulation* 32(1):139–149.

Vila-Badia, R., A. Butjosa, N. Del Cacho, C. Serra-Arumi, M. Esteban-Sanjusto, S. Ochoa, and J. Usall. 2021. Types, prevalence and gender differences of childhood trauma in first-episode psychosis. What is the evidence that childhood trauma is related to symptoms and functional outcomes in first episode psychosis? A systematic review. *Schizophrenia Research* 228:159–179.

Walker, D. L., K. J. Ressler, K. T. Lu, and M. Davis. 2002. Facilitation of conditioned fear extinction by systemic administration or intra-amygdala infusions of D-cycloserine as assessed with fear-potentiated startle in rats. *Journal of Neuroscience* 22(6):2343–2351.

Westerman, H. B., G. L. Suarez, L. S. Richmond-Rakerd, R. Nusslock, K. L. Klump, S. A. Burt, and L. W. Hyde. 2024. Exposure to community violence as a mechanism linking neighborhood socioeconomic disadvantage and neural responses to reward. *Social Cognitive and Affective Neuroscience* 19(1):nsae029.

Wingo, A. P., G. Wrenn, T. Pelletier, A. R. Gutman, B. Bradley, and K. J. Ressler. 2010. Moderating effects of resilience on depression in individuals with a history of childhood abuse or trauma exposure. *Journal of Affective Disorders* 126(3):411–414.

Wrenn, K., B. Lorenzen, I. Jones, C. Zhou, and D. Aronsky. 2010. Factors affecting stress in emergency medicine residents while working in the ED. *Annals of Emergency Medicine* 28(8):897–902.

Writing Committee for the ENRICHD Investigators. 2003. Effects of treating depression and low perceived social support on clinical events after myocardial infarction. *Journal of the American Medical Association* 289:3106-3116.

Xia, F., V. Fascianelli, N. Vishwakarma, F. G. Ghinger, A. Kwon, M. M. Gergues, L. K. Lalani, S. Fusi, and M. A. Kheirbek. 2025. Understanding the neural code of stress to control anhedonia. *Nature* 637(8046):654–662.

Yeo, B. T., F. M. Krienen, J. Sepulcre, M. R. Sabuncu, D. Lashkari, M. Hollinshead, J. L. Roffman, J. W. Smoller, L. Zöllei. J. R. Polimeni, and B. Fischl. 2011. The organization of the human cerebral cortex estimated by intrinsic functional connectivity. *Journal of Neurophysiology* 106(3):1125-1165.

Zhang, T. Y., C. L. Keown, X. Wen, J. Li, D. A. Vousden, C. Anacker, U. Bhattacharyya, R. Ryan, J. Diorio, N. O'Toole, J. P. Lerch, E. A. Mukamel, and M. J. Meaney. 2018. Environmental enrichment increases transcriptional and epigenetic differentiation between mouse dorsal and ventral dentate gyrus. *Nature Communications* 9(1):298.

Zhu, H., X. Yang, S. Xie, and J. Zhou. 2023. Prevalence of burnout and mental health problems among medical staff during the COVID-19 pandemic: A systematic review and meta-analysis. *BMJ Open* 13(7):e061945.

Appendix B

Workshop Agenda

APPLYING NEUROBIOLOGICAL INSIGHTS ON STRESS TO FOSTER RESILIENCE ACROSS THE LIFESPAN: A WORKSHOP

National Academy of Sciences Building
2101 Constitution Avenue, NW
Washington, DC 20418

MARCH 24, 2025
LECTURE ROOM

2:00–2:05	Introductory Remarks **Frances Jensen**, *University of Pennsylvania*; Co-chair, Forum on Neuroscience and Nervous System Disorders; Planning Committee Member **Deanna Barch**, *Washington University in St. Louis*; Co-chair, Forum on Neuroscience and Nervous System Disorders; Planning Committee Member **Margarita Alegría**, *Massachusetts General Hospital and Harvard Medical School*; Co-chair, Forum on Mental Health and Substance Use Disorders

2:05–2:10	Workshop Overview **Huda Akil**, *University of Michigan*, Workshop Co-chair
2:10–2:30	Keynote Presentation: State of Science on Stress and Resilience **Huda Akil**, *University of Michigan*, Workshop Co-chair
2:30–2:40	A Lived-Experience Perspective on Resilience **Jon Nelson**, *Pulverize the Stigma*

SESSION 1—NEUROBIOLOGICAL MECHANISMS OF STRESS SUSCEPTIBILITY AND RESILIENCE

- Review scientific evidence on the global rise of stress, disparities among populations, and the relationship between stress and development of systemic disorders (e.g., psychiatric, neurological, metabolic, cardiovascular, autoimmune), highlighting specific examples.

2:40–2:45	Session Overview **Aleksandra Vicentic** (virtual), *National Institute of Mental Health*, Planning Committee Member **Michael Milham**, *Child Mind Institute*, Planning Committee Member
2:45–2:55	**Scott Russo**, *Icahn School of Medicine at Mount Sinai*
2:55–3:05	**Mazen Kheirbek**, *University of California, San Francisco*
3:05–3:15	**Michael Baratta**, *University of Colorado*
3:15–3:35	BREAK
3:35–4:00	**Judy Cameron**, *University of Pittsburgh* **Kerry Ressler**, *McLean Hospital and Harvard Medical School*
4:00–4:45	Moderated Panel and Audience Q&A

4:45–5:00 Day 1 Concluding Remarks
Huda Akil, *University of Michigan*, Workshop Co-chair
Eric Nestler, *Icahn School of Medicine at Mount Sinai*, Workshop Co-chair

5:00 Adjourn Day 1

MARCH 25, 2025
LECTURE ROOM

9:30 Review of Day 1 and Preview of Day 2
Huda Akil, *University of Michigan*, Workshop Co-chair
Eric Nestler, *Icahn School of Medicine at Mount Sinai*, Workshop Co-chair

9:40 A Lived-Experience Perspective on Resilience
Indida Birto, *Here's to Life*

SESSION 2—PERIODS OF OPPORTUNITY FOR RESILIENCE AND ADAPTIVE NEUROPLASTICITY ACROSS THE LIFESPAN

- Examine recent discoveries illuminating the neurobiological mechanisms of stress susceptibility, distinct mechanisms of resilience, and individual differences in responses to stress and building resilience.

9:50–9:55 Session Overview
Brian Dias, *University of Southern California*, Planning Committee Member
Frances Jensen, *University of Pennsylvania*, Planning Committee Member

9:55–10:05 **Catherine Jensen Peña**, *Princeton University*, Planning Committee Member

10:05–10:15 **Michael Meaney**, *McGill University*

10:15–10:25 **Cynthia Rogers**, *Washington University in St. Louis*

10:25–10:35 **Luke Hyde**, *University of Michigan* (virtual)

10:35–10:45 **Darby Saxbe**, *University of Southern California* (virtual)

10:55–11:30 Moderated Panel and Audience Q&A

11:30–11:45 BREAK

SESSION 3—SYSTEMIC MANIFESTATIONS AND OUTCOMES OF STRESS SUSCEPTIBILITY AND RESILIENCE

- Consider the role of childhood neurodevelopment and neuroplasticity across the lifespan in building early life and lifelong resilience (as opposed to stress susceptibility) and discuss effective approaches for optimizing resilience during critical and sensitive periods of neurodevelopment.

11:45–11:55 Session Overview
Deanna Barch, *Washington University in St. Louis*; Co-chair, Forum on Neuroscience and Nervous System Disorders; Planning Committee Member
John Krystal, *Yale University*, Planning Committee Member

11:55–12:05 **Janitza Montalvo-Ortiz**, *Yale University*

12:05–12:15 **Tamar Gur**, *Ohio State University*

12:15–12:25 **J. Douglas Bremner**, *Emory University*

12:25–1:00 Moderated Panel and Audience Q&A

1:00–1:45 LUNCH BREAK

SESSION 4—CLINICAL AND PUBLIC HEALTH INTERVENTIONS

- Explore how these findings could inform public health programs and education to promote resilience to stress.

1:45–1:50 Session Overview
Andrew Fuligni, *University of California, Los Angeles*, Planning Committee Member

	Husseini Manji, *Oxford University*, *Yale University*, Planning Committee Member
1:50–2:00	**Nadine Burke Harris**, *ACE Resource Network*, Planning Committee Member
2:00–2:10	**Velma McBride Murry**, *Vanderbilt University*
2:10–2:20	**Helen Minnis**, *University of Glasgow* (virtual)
2:25–3:00	Moderated Panel and Audience Q&A
3:00–3:15	BREAK

SESSION 5—SYNTHESIS AND OPPORTUNITIES FOR PROMOTING RESILIENCE

- Discuss research gaps and opportunities for studying resilience across research, clinical, and public settings.

3:15–3:20	Session Overview **Eric Nestler**, *Icahn School of Medicine at Mount Sinai*, Workshop Co-chair
3:20–3:55	Themes and Future Opportunities Discussion **Frances Jensen**, *University of Pennsylvania*; Co-chair, Forum on Neuroscience and Nervous System Disorders; Planning Committee Member **John Krystal**, *Yale University*, Planning Committee Member **Husseini Manji**, *Oxford University*, *Yale University*, Planning Committee Member **Jon Nelson**, *Pulverize the Stigma* **Aleksandra Vicentic**, *National Institute of Mental Health*, Planning Committee Member (virtual)
3:55–4:00	Concluding Remarks **Huda Akil**, *University of Michigan*, Workshop Co-chair **Eric Nestler**, *Icahn School of Medicine at Mount Sinai*, Workshop Co-chair
4:00	Adjourn Day 2